B.S.A.V.A

MANUAL OF LABORATORY TECHNIQUES

(New Edition)

Edited by

D. L. Doxey
B.V.M.&S., Ph.D., M.R.C.V.S.

and

M. B. F. Nathan
M.A., B.V.Sc., M.R.C.V.S.

Published by
British Small Animal
Veterinary Association
5 St. Georges Terrace
Cheltenham
Glos. GL50 3PT

Printed by KCO, Worthing
West Sussex

Published 1989

ISBN 0 905214 08 0

CONTENTS

CONTENTS

CONTENTS

CONTENTS

ACKNOWLEDGEMENTS

I would like to thank all the contributors for their enthusiasm in helping to produce, this, the third edition of the manual. In particular acknowledgement must be made to Dr. David Doxey who has been responsible for scrutinising the scientific content of the papers. My thanks, too, to Michael Gorton Design for the graphics, and coping with an extremely tight schedule. The publication has been designed for the practising Veterinary Surgeon and is not intended as an in depth work of reference.

MICHAEL NATHAN
Damory Veterinary Clinic, Blandford, Dorset

AUTHORS

J. ARMOUR, Ph.D., M.R.V.S.
University of Glasgow

P. J. BROWN, B.V.M.S., Ph.D., M.R.C.V.S.
University of Bristol

H. J. C. CORNWELL, B.V.M.S., Ph.D.
University of Glasgow

D. L. DOXEY, B.V.M.&S., Ph.D., M.R.C.V.S.
University of Edinburgh

M. P. FLEMING, M.I.Biol., S.R.M.L.S.,
Vetlab Services

D. R. E. JONES, M.Sc., Ph.D., F.I.M.L.S.
University of Stirling

M. G. KERR, B.V.M.S., BSc., M.R.C.V.S.
Verlab Services

G. H. K. LAWSON, B.V.M.&S., B.Sc., Ph.D., M.R.C.V.S.
University of Edinburgh

G. S. WALTON, B.V.Sc., M.R.C.V.S.
University of Liverpool

FOREWORD

This manual has been rewritten in the majority and the content of the second edition has been greatly augmented. There are two new chapters on virology and immunology, and expansion of the section on clinical chemistry by the separate consideration of Urine Analysis, and Transudates and Exudates. Chapter one has been rewritten to reflect the needs, capabilities and costs of setting up a practice laboratory. It is thought provoking and to be recommended.

The improvements reflect the rapid rise and demand for reliable diagnostic backup, interpretative accompanying information and an understanding of sophisticated techniques and equipment. This last year has seen an unprecedented demand by practices to set up their own laboratories against the background of even greater diversity and complexity of tests being performed for them by an enhanced number of commercial laboratories.

The engine for this change has to be the familiarity of the use of laboratory tests and education on the subject both of new graduates and established practitioners coupled with a general awareness of diagnostic values.

On the one hand is the demand for acute diagnosis; the sick animal is defined by clinical examination and its problem refined by clinical pathology. But on the other hand there has been a marked awareness of the need for preventive medicine, even in the small animal field. Practices now run obesity clinics, geriatric clinics, and routine period or yearly health checks all of which have a greater and greater potential for the use of laboratory and other 'side-room' techniques.

Greater knowledge on what can be done, fuels dissemination of information on what should be done. Public demand awakened by this as well as the ability to afford resultant fees whether because of greater disposable income or health insurance or both provides the practitioner with even more scope to develop latent skills.

The caveat to this explosion of demand is well borne out in this book, however. The advantages of an in-house laboratory facility are legion. Postal delays and loss are avoided. The speed of results does not need to be sold to anyone and the consequent illustration of the practice's skills and in-depth service are excellent PR. On the other hand the facility is labour intensive, requires well trained staff with great integrity and a throughput of material sufficient to ensure accuracy from familiarity with techniques through to the improvement of cost-effectiveness.

This manual is designed for instant and yet studied reference. It stresses the need to realise that the quality of the result is equal to the quality of the sample taken and received. Haemolysis in serum, incorrect media or bad packaging, and inappropriate sampling conditions will obliterate the chance for a significant and reliable answer.

It stresses the need for careful thought and consideration before each and every action, from the setting up of the laboratory to the selection of the sample container, and promotes an understanding as to why one and not the other.

It stresses the need for care, not just of operator integrity, but for the health and safety of the worker in this increasingly hazardous area.

S. J. FOSTER, B.V.Sc., Cert.V.Ophthal., M.R.C.V.S.
President B.S.A.V.A.

CHAPTER 1

ESTABLISHING AND RUNNING A PRACTICE LABORATORY

M. P. Fleming M.I.Biol., S.R.L.M.S.

INTRODUCTION

Currently, veterinary practices in the United Kingdom are spoilt for choice as regards the number of commercial veterinary laboratories available to which specimens can be sent. Service from this source has been steadily improving and become more professional over the last few years. Some now offer veterinary interpretations and advice with their results. Clearly this needs to be considered carefully before deciding to establish one's own laboratory, especially if the commercial laboratory is close by and/or runs a free specimen collection service.

At this point it may be useful to enumerate the advantages of using a practice laboratory, which are:-

1.   Potential for faster results.
2.   Potential for more accurate results on perishable samples.
3.   Potential to use laboratory tests more frequently.
4.   Potential to have direct control over accuracy and speed of results.
5.   Potential to decrease cost of tests.
6.   Potential to increase practice profits.
7.   Potential to select test of own choice.
8.   Potential to improve client relations and practice image.
9.   Elimination of packing and posting specimens.
10.   Elimination of postal delays.
11.   Elimination of damage to or loss of specimens in post.
12.   Elimination of having to telephone laboratory for results.

From this list it is apparent that the number of advantages of having one's own laboratory shrinks considerably if a commercial veterinary laboratory is nearby and specimens can be delivered there the same day. Clearly, having anything other than a small scale laboratory would be difficult to justify in this case. Having decided to establish or expand your own practice laboratory, there are several areas you must consider.

CRITERIA FOR SUCCESS

Most practices do not have the luxury of having a nearby veterinary laboratory and thus will still be attracted by the **potential** advantages of having their own. In order to be reasonably sure that these potential benefits can actually be achieved, it is wise to consider the practice's ability to fulfil the following criteria:

Familiarity with tests

Most, if not all, the veterinary staff should be thoroughly familiar with the tests offered. This includes when to request them and what the results mean. This is a very obvious pre-requisite but one which is frequently overlooked by practices who are used to relying on commercial laboratories for this information.

Adequate veterinary supervision and staff training

At least one enthusiastic, technically experienced, veterinary surgeon should be responsible for the establishing and running of the laboratory. He/she will need to liaise closely with all other staff, supervise laboratory staff and train them, and be responsible for the accuracy and reliability of results produced. He/she will also need to be capable of interpreting results and possibly assisting colleagues in this area. More details on the veterinary supervisor's duties are given in the sections on 'Staffing and Training'. This position is of vital importance to the successful running of any practice laboratory. Laboratory staff must have a desire to work in the laboratory, appropriate educational attainments and be given a sense of responsibility.

Sufficient demand for tests

There has to be adequate demand for individual tests otherwise it is not cost-effective or efficient to process them in a laboratory. Each test has to be considered separately, remembering that in most cases if a particular test is undertaken on more than one specimen at a time the direct cost per test is considerably reduced. One also has to consider the frequency with which tests are done, not only from the cost point of view, but regular testing is often necessary to maintain the required level of skill. It is best to start by considering the current frequency of samples sent away and the tests requested by the practice. Could there be any increase if done in-house and if so, what would the frequency be? Having arrived at a final figure per week for each test, one must then thoroughly research the direct costs, overheads, and labour costs which will be involved. If tests are relatively simple and quick to perform these costs will be minimised.

Time

Most practice tests take a significant amount of time to complete thoroughly and conscientiously, and staff must not be hurried or asked to do other tasks as well. Remember that time must not only be allowed to do the test but also to gather together reagents and equipment, start up instruments, and also run calibration and quality control checks. Finally, test results have to be recorded, possibly on two forms. All this may mean the loss of a trainee nurse for at least half of the week. Please also ensure that staff know when they will be expected to work in the laboratory well in advance. It is good to agree on a set period each day and if no specimens appear it can always be agreed that they do something else.

Space

Every laboratory must have sufficient space and be quiet. Laboratory work demands thoroughness and intense concentration. Lack of space promotes untidiness and a cluttered bench often promotes a cluttered mind. Noise will also cause lack of concentration. Both lead to mistakes such as sample results being mixed up or forgotten to be recorded, erroneous results, and tests having to be re-run because of missing timed steps in a procedure.

Finance

Capital will be required to purchase equipment, furnishings and initial stocks of reagents and consumables. Labour costs must also be considered as well as other general overheads.

Clearly, all of the above criteria are important, but some more than others. I believe that I have listed them in order of importance but would stress again the importance of staff. It is very common for practices to fail in this area and the laboratory, if set up, usually fails miserably.

ACTIVITY PLAN

This will simply consist of a list of tests that will be routinely performed in the practice laboratory. This will, however, be influenced by many inter-related factors such as their relevance to the species of animal seen by the practice and the six criteria for success previously listed. As a guide, suggestions for three different levels of practice laboratory are shown in Table 1.1 together with equipment and staff required. More details concerning the specific pieces of equipment needed in each test will be given in subsequent chapters, but the total costs given are accurate at the time of going to press and include all reagent and consumable costs. An accurate number of staff required cannot be given, of course, because this is largely influenced by workload, although what matters more is the quality of staff available. The activity plan is extremely important as it will greatly influence the initial design of the laboratory.

Table 1.1
Activity plan for three levels of practice laboratory.

Level	Test/procedure	Equipment and Cost	Staff
1.	Urine chemistry Serum/plasma separation PCV Plasma protein Urine S.G. Blood glucose Blood urea	Centrifuge (dual purpose) PCV reader Refractometer(dual purpose) Test strips Other (glucometer) **cost £650**	One or two trainee nurses in spare time
2.	**as level 1 plus:** Urine sediment Calculus analysis Parasitology Trypsin & smear Total WBC (Differential WBC) FeLV (Blood chemistry)	**as level 1 plus:** Microscope Water bath Haemocytometer Pipettor 0.1 — 1.0 ml Pipettor 50µl McMaster chamber Other (Reflectance photometer) **cost £1,600** **(cost £3,500 — £4,500)**	Fully lab. trained veterinary nurse with at least one assistant. Moderate degree of skill required (except for diff. WBC which requires special training).
3.	**as level 2 plus:** R.B.C. count Haemoglobin Platelet count Differential WBC Full blood chemistry Dermatophyte culture (Bacteriology)	**as level 2 plus:** Photometer Pipettor 10µl — 30µl Other Haematology Analyser Incubator 37°C Incubator 27°C **cost £6,000** **(cost £4,600)**	Full or part-time Technician/s or very experienced V. N. with assistants. Technician experienced in veterinary diagnostic bacteriology essential.

Note: Bracketed tests could be added at that level either by buying extra equipment or with additional technical skills, details of which have also been bracketed. Minor items, such as paper towels, are not included on the lists.

LABORATORY DESIGN

Position

The laboratory should ideally be in a position free from all external noise, through traffic and any other form of distraction, yet still remain readily accessible to veterinary and other staff.

Any form of distraction must be avoided because the work demands intense concentration and staff will not be able to do their job properly otherwise. This includes the elimination of other staff passing through the laboratory work area, the telephone, situations close to road traffic, kennelled animals or a busy office or waiting room.

Accessibility of the laboratory may mean a situation close to the consulting room(s) and at least on the same floor level. This helps to avoid the need for a telephone (a nuisance when one is in the middle of a fiddly test) and useful when an urgent test is required quickly e.g. whilst the client waits.

The laboratory should also be close to toilet facilities and separate rest/tea room and cloakroom. Ideally, it should also be situated on an outside wall with glass windows to allow daylight to enter and staff to see out. Whilst this greatly enhances morale it is not vital, however. If there is a choice of rooms a situation close to essential services especially water pipes and drains and electricity supply, will be preferred as will a room with two doors instead of one for safety reasons.

Space

This will be needed for benching (with cupboards underneath), a large refrigerator (not under bench), storage of some bulky consumables, filing cabinet, bookcase, desk, chairs, a separate wash hand basin and an area to hang laboratory coats as well as space to move around in.

Activities and workload will largely dictate exactly how much space is required. Common areas of activity in any practice laboratory include specimen receipt and preparation for testing, despatch of specimens to outside laboratories, recording/labelling/reporting procedures and ordering, all of which will need at least 2 metres of bench space and probably space for a desk and filing cabinet.

Bearing all this in mind, a level 1 laboratory (see Table 1.1) will therefore require at least six square metres. It could share space with some other facility, such as a store, as long as essential services were available and there were no distractions. Levels 2 and 3 laboratories, however, ought to be self-contained units with level 2 laboratory having at least 12 square metres of space.

One of the most significant factors influencing space in these laboratories is the range of tests provided. Generally each category of test or discipline (e.g. biochemistry, haematology) will require its own area of bench space (at least two metres) so that the appropriate reagents and equipment can be positioned readily to hand. This helps speed up testing and avoids confusion and untidiness when two or more people may need to work in the laboratory.

Workload has little immediate impact on space required, especially bench space but, as it increases, a point will be reached where two or more people may need to work in the laboratory at the same time and this will demand more room to move.

The Floor

This should be level and capable of bearing considerable weight, a factor which must be considered if sited on a first or second floor. The best materials are linoleum or vinyl sheeting which should be treated with a non-slip sealant (a type of polish) to improve cleaning and maximise life. The floor should be cleaned at least once a week.

Benches and Storage

The two options open to a practice are either kitchen units (Texas Home Stores, B & Q, Payless etc) or custom made benching with or without cupboards built in. Many practices have used the former with great success and they can be recommended provided they are not required to support items in excess of about 20—30 lbs. Custom made benching has the advantage of being built to personal specifications, especially height (see later), is self supporting allowing easy movement of under bench storage units and will support weighty items of equipment.

In any case, a comfortable height for a bench top is 0.88—0.98 metres and width of 0.6—0.7 metres, where the bench runs alongside a wall, or 1.2—1.5 metres for a two-sided (peninsular) bench. The bench top itself should be rigid and covered in a plastic laminate with a minimum of joints. The choice of colour is personal but light colours enhance the decor and help morale, whilst dark colours hide the stains (and dirt) and provide a convenient background against which certain tests can be viewed e.g. slide agglutinations, culture plate reading.

Before purchasing benching in any form it is wise to draw a plan of the laboratory showing the area to be benched including positioning of sinks and under bench storage units. It is, however, important to allow space under benches for kneeholes where staff have to sit and the possibility of storing boxes of bulky consumables. One advantage of having a bench top height of 0.98 metres is that staff can stand and work at it as well as sit. This cuts down the number of kneeholes required, and increases under bench storage space. Having finalised the layout plan, underbench cupboard and draw units can be purchased. Cupboard units should have shelves and sliding doors. It is not wise to use wall cupboards as they look unsightly and restrict air space over benches, although possibly this is a matter of opinion. Narrow shelving on walls over benches is a practical alternative as long as they are kept tidy. A refrigerator will also be required and the bigger the better because as a laboratory grows so does its demand for fridge space. A free standing refrigerator of about 4' 6'' high with freezer compartment will be invaluable, as will a filing cabinet to store records and suppliers details.

Heating, Lighting and Ventilation

It is essential to have some form of heating as some tests are designed to work at 'room temperature' as are certain types of equipment. Also, staff will not be performing tests correctly if they are cold. Storage radiators, oil-filled electric radiators or, ideally, water radiators, thermostatically controlled as part of the practice central heating system, are all suitable. Mobile gas cylinder fires are also effective but allow adequate ventilation and do not use them in the presence of inflammable liquids.

Natural ventilation, without draughts, is best but installation of one or two extractor fans can be useful. The opening of doors and windows in summer should be avoided if bacteriology and mycology culturing is performed.

Working at a bench in front of a window is good for morale although, if it faces south, blinds may be needed. In any case, adequate fluorescent lighting is essential as most tests require careful observation e.g. urine test strips.

Laboratory Services

Electricity. The best advice is to consult a qualified electrician and ask him to install the entire system. It is a necessary cost. He will advise on the number of electrical circuits required, circuit breakers, earthing and positioning of fuse box as well as ensuring proper installation. All laboratories rely heavily on electricity and it is wise to plan for as many electrical outlets as possible even if they are not required immediately. It is dangerous to use adaptors and inconvenient to continuously connect and disconnect instruments from the power supply.

Electrical outlets should not be placed near sinks or any other area where liquids are likely to be spilt. They should be postitioned on walls about six inches from the bench surface or, if on a peninsular or island bench, mounted on a plinth in the centre at an angle of at least 45 degrees.

Water. At the time of drawing the layout plan of the laboratory, a plumber should be consulted or at least the whereabouts of the water mains and drainage known. Sinks will have to be planned as near to these services as possible in order to minimise installation costs.

A cold water supply and at least two sinks are required in most laboratories, one for hand-washing and the other for stains, solution preparation and harmless liquid waste disposal. Again, I would advise consulting and engaging a professional to do the job. Cold water can be heated by using an electric water heater at the hand basin (a job for the electrician, also).

Gas. This is not really necessary for most practice laboratories except those who do bacteriology and fungal culture. If only a few cultures are done then a small camping gas fire using a cylinder is sufficient, or the same cylinder with a bunsen burner attachment. If more work is done a proper system may need to be installed connected to North Sea gas or Calor gas cylinders.

BASIC EQUIPMENT

A list of all the equipment likely to be required in any practice laboratory is shown in Table 1.1, whilst more detailed information about any item of specialised equipment will be found in the appropriate chapter in this book. However, it is worth mentioning something about the following general purpose instruments.

Centrifuge

This is the first item that any practice will buy. However, it needs to be a dual-purpose centrifuge, one that will perform microhaematocrits as well as centrifuge whole blood samples for serum or plasma and ideally both functions should be performed in the same rotor. Therefore the centrifuge must be capable of at least 11,000 rpm, have a timer control, and a rotor which will accept both microhaematocrit capillaries and tubes of at least 1.5 ml capacity or more. To the best of my knowledge the only two centrifuges available in the U.K. that fulfill these criteria are the 'Selectafuge' available from BCL Ltd.

and the 'Hawksley Combination Centrifuge' available from Vetlab Services. Both instruments have a proven track record as regards reliability and are supported by an excellent repairs service. Both instruments can also be used to centrifuge other items like urine but when used to do this, or centrifuge blood tubes, the rotor must be balanced with a tube of liquid of equal volume directly opposite the sample otherwise dangerous vibrations will result. No balancing is required, however, when performing microhaematocrits.

Microscope

This will be required for levels 2 and 3 practice laboratories. One should not buy anything other than a binocular model with built-in illumination, a rheostat-controlled light source, adjustable condenser, and a mechanical stage. A set of good quality achromat objectives of x4, x10 and x40 magnification together with x10 eyepiece lenses, for faecal and hair parasitology, urine sediments, faecal smears, total w.b.c. and r.b.c counts and dermatophyte spore detection, together with x10 eyepiece lenses, should also be purchased. An oil immersion objective of x100 will also be required for cytology, blood smears and Gram-stained smears. It is vital that these objectives and the whole system is of good optical quality, the critical test being the image achieved at a total magnification of x1000. It is also useful for the microscope to be capable of updating with flat-field objectives, wide field eye piece lenses (a boon for the haematology technician reading blood smears), and photographic equipment. Rubber eye guards for eyepiece lenses are also popular. A good microscope, cared for correctly, will last at least 10 or 15 years or even more. It is an extremely valuable diagnostic tool on a par with an X-ray or anaesthetic machine. Unfortunately, most veterinarians do not think of it in this way and tend to want to buy the cheapest microscope available. Whilst price is important, a quality instrument that facilitates microscope diagnosis and requires little maintainance provides a much better return on investment than a cheaper one. I know of at least twenty cases where practices have finally had to buy good microscopes to replace their 'cheap' monocular models, and the delight expressed when they were 'seeing things they had never seen before'! Laboratory staff also tend to be impressed by an employer who thinks in this way and tend to work better in return.

Finally, it should be stressed that, whilst the maintenance of microscopes is minimal, care must be taken to keep them clean and in particular microscope oil should **always** be wiped off oil-immersion lenses after use. If not, oil will eventually seep up inside the objective and may ruin the lens.

Refractometer

The 'pocket' version of this instrument is extremely simple to operate and essential for accurate urine specific gravity measurement. I would advise that one is purchased with a dual scale for urine specific gravity **and** serum or plasma total protein. The latter test can be performed on a small drop of serum or plasma either from a centrifuged blood tube or from the plasma layer after reading a microhaematocrit capillary. The tube is snapped above the packed erythrocyte layer and plasma allowed to run out onto the prism of the refractometer.

Finally, it should be emphasised that all laboratory equipment requires correct operation and maintenance. The veterinary supervisor must ensure that laboratory staff and himself/herself fully understand, not only the maintenance and operation procedures, but also the principle involved. It is wise, on the receipt of any new instrument, to take the manual home, study it from cover to cover and when fully familiar with it, prepare one's own user guide as a precis of the manufacturer's. It is important that this is kept as simple as possible and that all procedures are described in simple, single steps. By doing this, not only does it aid familiarity with the instrument, but photocopies of operation and maintenance procedures can also be pinned to the wall next to the instrument for all to see. It is important in this document to stress the frequency of each maintenance and calibration procedure as this is all too frequently forgotten. To ensure these are carried out, a log book should be provided for all staff to record when and what was done, and to record any faults. This is extremely useful in helping to diagnose faults, saving unnecessary frustration and service engineers' bills. On this point, when an instrument is out of warranty, it is advisable to purchase a service contract from the manufacturer especially if the instrument is used heavily and generating profits. Such contracts may be expensive and should not be entered into without due consideration.

STAFFING AND TRAINING

It is essential that one member of the veterinary staff has overall responsibility for the laboratory. He/she (the veterinary supervisor) will then be in a position to liaise with the other veterinary staff and likely to have some influence on decisions affecting the running and expansion of the laboratory. He/she will also be in an ideal situation to assess the usefulness, accuracy and efficiency of the laboratory, not only from his/her own clinical point of view, but also from that of the other veterinary staff. The veterinary supervisor will require an assistant (the lab. assistant) who will actually work in the laboratory. In a level 1 laboratory this will probably be either a veterinary nurse or trainee but as the laboratory gets larger this position will be filled by a trained technician. The lab. assistant will have had thorough training in all tests performed either from previous experience, or in-house training by the veterinary supervisor or from an outside laboratory that offers training courses. The position will also involve training other assistants who will cover in emergencies, sickness and holidays, and ordering/stock control as well as performing and reporting the tests.

Both the veterinary supervisor and the lab. assistant need to communicate frequently with each other. The former must be able to get on with his/her clinical duties but at the same time keep a careful eye on the accuracy and speed of results being produced. In order to do this it is necessary for at least weekly meetings to be held for two-way communication **without interruption**. The lab. assistant will look to the veterinary supervisor for support and feedback. For example a good lab. assistant/technician will greatly appreciate a comment such as 'You were right. That high WBC count and left shift you reported on Mr. Brown's dog turned out to be a pyometra and your results helped me to operate just in time. Well done!' The observation is an indirect means of quality control and the communication a very effective way of improving morale. In the same way it is also a good idea to teach laboratory staff the significance of laboratory results as it helps them to help you better. For example, they will appreciate why you want the blood urea done urgently or that you will want to know immediately about a blood glucose level of 27 mmol/litre.

On the other hand the veterinary supervisor will be looking for an assistant that can be trusted not only to do the tests correctly and quickly, but someone with an enquiring mind who asks questions and who can spot mistakes. One of the hallmarks of a good technician is the ability to check and double check procedures during the test and results afterwards for any errors. They therefore must have the qualities of thoroughness, conscientiousness, keenness and intelligence. In my experience, any person being considered for a trainee laboratory assistant/technician position will only be successful if in possession of a least 4 or 5 good 'O' level passes including Maths, Chemistry and Physics or Biology. If they prove successful one can help further their career by offering to send them on a part-time BTEC course in Biological Sciences at a local college, an offer which should be greatly appreciated and at least help to ensure they remain with the practice for several more years.

Finally, one must ensure that adequate numbers of staff are available to do the tests, not only during normal working hours, but afterwards as well. This may involve training many more staff than would actually work routinely in the laboratory, including veterinary staff. Always bear in mind that staff can be sent to other laboratories for training especially if one is friendly with someone there. Thus it pays to maintain as many contacts in outside laboratories as possible, and definitely not wise to cut off any commercial laboratory to whom you were originally sending samples, completely.

SAMPLE AND REPORT PROCESSING

Request/report form.

It is essential to have written instructions concerning the tests required supplied with a specimen and also a form on which the results are recorded. It is therefore sensible to combine all this information on just one form (see Figure 1.1).

The top portion will need to contain the following information: Veterinary Surgeon, owner's name and address, animal's name, date of sampling, species, age, sex, specimen description, clinical signs and differential diagnosis. The last two pieces of information are necessary from the clinician's point of view to remind him/her of this vital information whilst reviewing the results, and to encourage laboratory staff's interest rather than treat them purely as number generators.

Figure 1.1
Example of practice laboratory request/report form.

VETERINARY PRACTICE
LABORATORY REQUEST / REPORT FORM

Date Sent	Lab. Ref. No.
Date Completed	

Species .... Breed ....Age .... Sex.........

Sample(s) ....

Clinical History and Diff Diagnosis ....

....

....

....

Owner ....

Address ....

....

Vet. Surg ....

BIOCHEMISTRY (at least 2ml heparinised blood please)

☐ Total Protein .... g/l   ☐ GGT .... u/l (37°C)   ☐ Magnesium ...... mmol/l

☐ Albumin................ g/l   ☐ CK .... u/l (37°C)   ☐ Calcium .... mmol/l

☐ Urea .... mmol/l   ☐ AST .... u/l (37°C)   ☐ Phosphate .... mmol/l

☐ Creatinine .... mmol/l   ☐ Glucose .... mmol/l   ☐ Selenium .... Units

☐ ALT............ u/l (37°C)   ☐ Bilirubin .... mmol/l   ☐ Copper .... mmol/l

☐ ALP............ u/l (37°C)   ☐ Cholesterol .... mmol/l   ☐ BHB .... mmol/l

☐ Urine Strip tests: pH .... S.G. .... Other positive findings ....

☐ Urine Sediment/Calculus analysis ....

HAEMATOLOGY (at least 1.0ml EDTA blood please).

☐ PCV ....

Plasma: N/lysed/jaundice/lipaemic

Plasma Protein ....

☐ Visual assessment of smear ....

....

....

☐ FeLV ....

☐ Total WBC .... x 10^9/l

☐ Differential WBC count

Neutrophils: adult ...... % .... x 10^9/l

band ..... % .... x 10^9/l

Eosinophils .... % .... x 10^9/l

Lymphocytes .... % .... x 10^9/l

Monocytes .... % .... x 10^9/l

PARASITOLOGY/TRYPSIN

☐ Faecal concentration (small animals) ....

☐ Worm Egg Count .... e.p.g.   ☐ Trypsin ....

☐ Baermann's ....   Smear ....

☐ Microscopy...................   Tech'n .... Date ....

☐ **SEND AWAY**

Sample...........................   Tests required...........................

Laboratory .... Date sent .... Date completed ....

Results ....

....

.... TOTAL FEE ....

In the main body of the form can be listed all the specific types of test offered grouped into the main disciplines: urine analysis, blood chemistry, haematology and parasitology. Each specific test name can be preceded by a box to be ticked when requested and a space allowed after the test name in which to record the result.

At the bottom of the form a category for sub-contracted test information can be provided together with price, date completed and technician's name. A form like this can easily be typewritten and either photocopied or printed as single sheets or in N.C.R. sets.

Sample and Form Handling

A completed form should arrive in the laboratory in some way attached to the specimen or at least all specimens should be labelled with the owner's name (hopefully, samples will not appear from two different owners with the same name at the same time!). The best method is to label all containers with owner's name and animal's name, and possibly tests required at sampling, and place inside one side of two-compartmented bag. The form can be folded and placed inside the other pouch and both will remain together until arrival in the laboratory. In the laboratory the type of specimen and the information written on their label should be checked with that written on the accompanying form to ensure no specimen/form mix up at this or any subsequent stage. In this respect it is also wise to buy some plastic trays inside which forms can be stacked with their specimens one set on top of another if a number of specimens and forms builds up.

Submission Processing Systems.

There are three main options:

Option 1 Place form and specimen on the appropriate part of the bench according to tests requested, do tests, record results direct on form, check, photocopy and despatch original. File copies either in date order or alphabetical order of owner's name.

Option 2 Transfer essential details from top section of form and tests required to a page of a **day book** (Figure 2) ruled with headed columns. Such information will probably be date, owner's name, animal's name, species and test required. Test required can be indicated by either ticking a narrow column within a test column or by marking the result area with a fluorescent yellow marker. Tests are then run and results immediately recorded in the day book, over the yellow marks if used. When all tests have been completed results are transferred to the original request/report forms which are checked, photocopied and despatched to the clinician.

Option 3 Transfer essential details from top section of form e.g. date, owner's and animal's names, specimen into an **entry book** and assign the entry a unique number. This number is then written on all specimen containers associated with the same case together with details of tests required. Alternatively, self-adhesive labels pre-printed with consecutive numbers can be obtained (Hughes and Hughes Ltd.) with sufficient space under the number to record test details in code. This number is also written on the top of the form or a label with the same number stuck to it. Now option 1 can be carried out or option 2 where the 'entry book' will actually need to be enlarged into a day book (Figure 1.2) or separate daybooks maintained for each discipline. (Figure 1.3).

Pros and cons. Option 1 is a very simple system for a laboratory handling very few specimens. One has to guard against the possibility of the form being taken before photocopying as this will leave the laboratory without a record. Reports are also liable to be messy, possibly with lots of 'Tippex' on. Otherwise a good simple system.

Option 2 has the following advantages.

a. Final reports usually neat and tidy.
b. A safeguard against lost copies of reports.
c. Faster recording of results in laboratory.
d. Results can quickly be accessed by any column heading e.g. owner or test result, especially if submission date known.

e. The results for a specific test, over a period of time, can quickly be assessed for any abnormal bias.

f. Statistical analyses can be easily performed e.g. daily workload easily assessed.

g. Outstanding tests obvious, reminding the technician to record results as soon as available.

And the disadvantages are:

a. More time consuming overall as results are recorded twice.

b. There is a limit to how many tests one can get on one page and the system relies on all entries on one sheet.

c. Reliance on handwritten owner's name as a means of identifying sample.

d. A problem may arise when two or more staff are performing different tests at the same time with only one day book.

Option 2 is, therefore, a more advanced system for laboratory dealing with more specimens but still with a limited range of tests — a level 2 practice laboratory, for example.

Option 3, combining an entry book and submission numbering system with Option 1, has worked well for me for up to 100 submissions a day. However, things become difficult if a submission requests test covering two or more disciplines in a laboratory where each discipline has its own staff and work is carried out simultaneously. Then there is only one form and the adoption of Option 2, using a separate daybook for each discipline, is advisable within Option 3.

I am reluctant to recommend a specific system for any set situation, rather suggest that each practice try all of them at some time and see which suits them.

Figure 1.2
Combined entry/day book for Level 1 practice laboratory.

SPECIMEN ENTRY BOOK					TEST DAY WORK SHEET								
					BLOOD			PLASMA		URINE			
Date	Lab. Ref.	Owner	Animal	Species	Gluco.	Urea	PCV	Colour	Protein	SG	pH	Other + ve	Send away
25/8/88	1010	SMITH	'FANG'	K9	22.0	8.5				1.010	6	—	
	1011	BLOGGS	'REX'	CAT		9.9	35	N	59				
	1012												

Figure 1.3
Separate day book for biochemistry using Lab. Ref. Numbers.

Date	Lab. Ref.	T.Prot.	Alb.	Urea	Creat.	ALT	ALP
25/8/88	Q.C. Range	47 – 55	30 – 36	8 – 10	185 – 200	38 – 48	56 – 70
	Q.C.	50	34	8.5	195	44	62
	1010	45	19				

It is advisable to perform each discipline on a separate area of bench. Thus, it may be useful to sort forms with their specimens into different trays according to type of test required, after entry of initial details, and deliver these to the appropriate bench areas.

Suitable categories/disciplines are obvious but when a submission covers more than one discipline the form and the specimen should go to the area of bench where results are likely to be finished first. If two or more people are working at the same time, but on different disciplines, the person who receives the form first must notify the other of any relevant test for them to perform. This is where a day book for each discipline becomes useful.

The above situation is a problem that can reasonably be coped with, but a much worse situation is when tests are requested in stages e.g. 'Do ALT and ALP. If normal, do PCV. If normal, do WBC'. This type of request, whilst obviously designed to economise, is really false economy especially in one's own laboratory. It will always lead to delay in a multi-discipline and staff laboratory where different disciplines are performed, and even in a small laboratory throws yet another trap for the unwary technician to fall into. It is more efficient to do a battery of tests all in one go, hence the popularity of profiles. After all, a negative or normal result is just as useful as a positive or abnormal one.

PROCEDURES FOR ASSURING QUALITY OF RESULTS

It is relatively easy to perform tests and produce results without checking their accuracy or precision (ability to produce the same result on repeat testings of the same sample). In fact, this is a common occurrence in small, busy laboratories especially where there is inconsistency in the staffing. It is also enhanced by the availability of seemingly fool-proof instruments and kits on the market which tempt the user into always trusting the results that are produced. The fact remains that laboratory procedures and instrumentation are very prone to Murphy's law which states that if anything can go wrong it will especially just when you don't want it to!

It is within this area, therefore, that the veterinary supervisor, together with the help of the lab. assistant, must start by laying down strict procedures for each test and the means by which its accuracy and precision will be measured. They must also constantly check that all these procedures are followed at all times and at the recommended frequency. There are also other more obvious ways of checking the accuracy of one's own laboratory tests which will be explained later.

1. **Test Manual**

   It is essential that procedures for all tests run in the laboratory are fully documented and available at all times to laboratory staff. Each procedure should be type-written on A4 paper and contain as much detail as possible including materials required, recipes for reagents, suppliers, principle of test procedure, actual procedure details broken down into single steps, how to read results and what they mean, what can go wrong and how to detect it, and quality control procedure. Each sheet of paper can be placed inside a plastic pocket/folder which can be clipped in an A4 ring binder. It may also be helpful to photocopy a procedure and fix it to the wall or other permanent fixture in the test area for easy reference.

2. **Instrument Manuals**

   Most manufacturers supply these but often they are difficult to understand or filled with a lot of detail which will not be routinely required. It is, therefore, a good idea to write one's own manual containing the bare essential operating, maintenance, calibration and quality control procedures. It is usually necessary to do this anyway, as the veterinary supervisor will have to decide on a strict policy concerning the frequency with which the last three procedures are carried out. To ensure that these instructions are carried out, a policy should be adopted of recording the results of these procedures, and/or the fact that they were carried out, in a **log book** which will be dated and signed. There is even more reason here to copy one's own instructions and display them on the wall by the instrument. It is good practice for all laboratory staff to be aware that an instrument must always be cleaned and/or calibrated, say, every Monday morning and that a log book will be maintained to check that this is done.

3. Direct Quality Control (Q.C.)

Strictly speaking, this is testing a sample or samples of known value. The principle is to check that the laboratory can produce accurate answers, but it is also a good idea to run these, or any other sample, at least four or five times to check also for precision. One important point to remember here is that the Q.C. sample's value should have been obtained using the method currently in use in the practice laboratory. Again the laboratory's policy concerning the time and frequency with which a Q.C. sample is run and the recording of its results must be made clear to all laboratory staff. For example 'Every Monday Q.C. samples A and B will be run for x,y, tests in triplicate and the results recorded in the log book' or 'The positive and negative control supplied in the kit must always be run with every batch of tests even a singleton'. The laboratory's policy on what to do if the Q.C. results are **not** what they should be, should also be made clear. Obviously the test results must not be reported and the veterinary supervisor consulted. A trained technician will know what to do but an inexperienced assistant may not.

Quality control samples are readily available for biochemistry and haematology but not for parasitology,mycology, urine analysis, faecal digestions or bacteriology. In the latter cases the problem may be overcome if contacts are available in the right places. For example, someone in the practice may know someone working in a parasitology department of a veterinary college who can send samples containing ova, mites etc. of known identity. Alternatively, the laboratory concerned might play host to the practice's technician and show them how to do things correctly. On this point commercial laboratories may also help and some will run training courses.

4. Quality Assurance (Q.A.).

This involves testing a sample whose results are unknown to staff. The results are then returned to an outside organiser and graded in relation to all the other laboratories participating in the scheme. This is only useful when large numbers of laboratories are involved. However, only schemes involving haematology, biochemistry and equine bacteriology are currently readily available for which a fee is charged.

It may not be practicable for a small practice laboratory to join such a scheme but the basic principles can easily be applied by the veterinary supervisor.

a . Split a sample and send one portion to a trustworthy laboratory. If it has to be posted then post your portion to yourself to allow for changes in transit. When comparing your results with the other laboratory's, check the method that they used as it may not give comparable results anyway.

b . Obtain a sample of known value from a friendly laboratory or a commercial Q.C. serum. Submit it to your laboratory as a sample (fake a request/report form). It is important not to tell the laboratory staff what it is as otherwise they will take abnormal care of it!

c . Use your clinical evaluation and that of your colleagues to check on your results. Is it picking up the renal failures, the pyometras, the anaemias and how do the results compare with the final clinical outcome of cases in general?

d . Request, or encourage the request, of tests which are interrelated e.g. haemoglobin, and PCV — if one is low all should be low (calculation of absolute values help here), or always run a creatinine if a blood urea is over 20 mmol/litre not only because of its diagnostic and prognostic value but also because a high urea with a normal creatinine, or vice versa, is most unusual and should be double checked.

5. Physical checking of written results.

Inexperienced staff often start by performing tests and recording results without thinking about anything else. I have even known such staff to record erroneous Q.C. results and report the test results which were run at the same time. Clearly, this is a matter of training but it is a good idea for the veterinary supervisor or some experienced staff member to check all reports before despatch for such things as: all tests requested have been done; agreement of inter-related test results and satisfactory absolute values; abnormal results which would be worth re-checking by re-testing the sample; decimal points in the right place; and anything else out of place. In addition, of course, the test results of all Q.C. samples run in parallel should be checked, and the overall trend of results examined in the day book e.g. why have all ALT results been low or normal recently, or why hasn't the laboratory been finding any parasite ova for the last 3 weeks? It is always encouraging to look at the day book and see highs, normals and lows or positives and negatives for each test scattered in the frequency one might expect, especially if the clinical history is displayed.

TROUBLESHOOTING

The previous section dealt with establishing a structure of correct procedure and alarm signals for when things go wrong. The next step is to know what to do when an alarm bell does ring. This is an area rarely appreciated by the average clinician wishing to set up his/her own laboratory (as is the area of Q.C.). For example, your checking procedures show that your laboratory has not detected helminth ova for the last 3 weeks and missed them in a known positive sample — what could be the cause and what can you do to confirm it? Or again, your Q.C. sample indicates persistent high results for creatinine together with imprecision — what do you do about it? Obviously, this is where having a trained technician with many years experience is a big advantage, but with inexperienced staff it could be a nightmare. Hence the reason for my placing bacteriology, blood chemistry and haematology in a level 3 laboratory where hopefully a trained technician will be available.

However, given a problem which the veterinary supervisor cannot solve using commonsense, one can often telephone a friendly laboratory or possibly the firm which supplied the instrumentation/reagents especially if that firm specialises in supplying veterinary practices. The latter may also offer to help even if the problem does not involve any of their products.

ORDERING/STOCK CONTROL

Obviously, a steady supply of consumables must be maintained without tying up a lot of money in stock. First, a duplicate book should be obtained from a stationers for use as an order book. The laboratory assistant will probably be in charge of ordering but this must be made clear, as should be the value to which items can be ordered without authorisation.

A list of all items required should then be compiled either in alphabetical order or in alphabetical order within various categories e.g. haematology, biochemistry, plastic consumables. These should be listed together with suppliers name, quantity usually ordered, price and usual delivery time. A separate list of suppliers details can be recorded in a box of record cards when one requires their telephone number, address or contact name. These details will be of immense value especially for comparing prices and checking suppliers invoices which is best done by the laboratory assistant.

At regular intervals all stock should be checked and/or all staff must be told to inform the laboratory assistant as soon as consumables get low. The problem is that a minimum or re-order stock level needs careful definition and equally the quantity to be ordered to top it up requires an experienced person's decision. Thus one person only should be responsible and it is best if they keep a constant watch on stocks rather than rely on others to tell them.

When ordering it is more efficient to post or fax written orders. Always specify acceptable delivery date especially on written orders and ask for notification if this cannot be achieved. Telephone only when orders are urgent, checking at the same time goods are in stock and always ask for the name of the person you are speaking to just in case you have to ring back or there is a mistake in the order. When ordering, ask for the delivery address to state 'The Laboratory' and ensure that other practice staff know where your parcels are to be placed otherwise your urgent parcel may get lost!

LABORATORY SAFETY

This is mainly commonsense but worth emphasising the main points.

1. No eating, smoking, drinking, biting fingernails, chewing the ends of pens or pencils or mouth pipetting for obvious reasons!

2. Protective white laboratory coats must be worn at all times except in the tea room.

3. Hands must be washed before leaving the laboratory for tea break, lunch or going home.

4. Strict attention must be given to waste disposal instructions, which should be displayed in the laboratory and definitely no needles, scalpel blades or glass in ordinary waste bins.

5. Strict attention must be given to recommended design of the laboratory, especially electric installations and adequate fire extinguishers should be supplied, especially of the carbon dioxide type for electrical fires. Always consult a professional electrician and your local fire department.

6. Bunsen burners must be turned off when not in use as their flame is sometimes invisible, especially in bright sunlight, and this can cause severe arm burns and singed hair!

7. Keep bench tidy at all times and enforce a policy of all benches having to be cleared and swabbed with disinfectant at the end of each day.

8. Immediately wipe up any liquid spilt on floor and ensure safe footwear (no high heels).

9. Maintain first aid kit in laboratory.

10. Provide laboratory staff with whatever specialised clothing is required. For example, rubber gloves or protective goggles.

11. All employees should read, understand and have available for perusal, information about the Health and Safety at Work Act 1974. Information relevant to Veterinary Practice can be found in the BVA publication 'Health and Safety at Work Act. A guide to veterinary practices 1978'.

CHAPTER 2

CLINICAL BIOCHEMISTRY

Morag. G. Kerr B.V.M.S., B.Sc., Ph.D., M.R.C.V.S.

INTRODUCTION

Appreciation of the usefulness of clinical biochemistry investigations is increasing continually. No matter how perceptive are one's clinical talents, it is impossible to come to a conclusive diagnosis in every single case on clinical grounds alone. While it is always possible to survive on a combination of retrospective diagnosis by assessing response to treatment and a good 'bedside manner', the addition of biochemical investigations to the diagnostic armoury cuts down on guesswork and allows a much more precise diagnosis to be made. This in turn improves patient care by allowing treatment regimes to be targeted to a known condition and, in particular, encourages perseverance with appropriate therapy even when the initial response appears disappointing.

Clinical biochemistry is particularly valuable because the patient itself and the state of its metabolism is being looked at, rather than other organisms which may (or may not) be responsible for the disease. The wide range of biochemical tests available mean that this discipline can provide information relating to a large number of different aspects of the patient's metabolism and allow a wide variety of conditions to be investigated. There should be no question, however, of using biochemistry tests as a substitute for clinical skills. On the contrary, sharp clinical acumen is essential in arriving at a reasonable provisional diagnosis and in judicial selection of the most appropriate tests to suit the circumstances — the laboratory investigations are an extension, not an alternative, to clinical examination and like all extensions, require to be built on a firm and well constructed base.

Once one is in the habit of using these investigations and is familiar with their potential, working in a practice where they are not available can feel disconcertingly like being required to examine patients blindfold and wearing sheepskin mittens. However, this is not a reflection of atrophied clinical skill, but the result of an awareness of the limitations of basic clinical methods and the extended possibilities which laboratory investigations offer.

SAMPLES

The required sample for most biochemical analyses is serum or heparinised plasma, with a strong preference for the latter so far as ease of processing is concerned. The only routine exception to this is that fluoride/oxalate plasma is required for glucose estimation.

Collection

The jugular vein is the site of choice, and the use of this vein is probably the most effective way of improving the quality of blood samples. The technique is shown in Figure 2.1; alternatively, cats or very small dogs may be restrained in lateral recumbency. Smaller, thin-walled veins (cephalic or saphenous) should be avoided wherever possible as the slow blood flow and tendency of the veins to collapse frequently results in haemolysed and/or clotted samples.

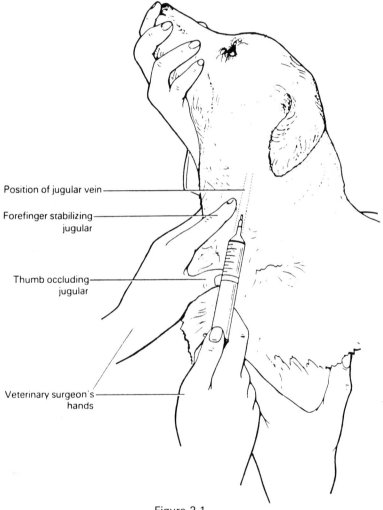

Position of jugular vein

Forefinger stabilizing jugular

Thumb occluding jugular

Veterinary surgeon's hands

Figure 2.1
Jugular blood collection in the dog

The most satisfactory technique is probably the syringe and the needle. Monovettes (both ordinary and 'safety') are also very good, but can be somewhat clumsy for small animal use. Vacutainers should be avoided whenever possible as the paediatric size produces very poor samples and the standard sizes tend to collapse small veins and to cause haemolysis. Dripping of blood from the end of a needle into a collection tube should also be avoided for both aesthetic reasons and because of the very poor quality of the samples obtained. Whichever method is used, it is very important to cap and mix all tubes with anticoagulant within a very few seconds after collection, otherwise clotting is extremely likely.

Processing

A large proportion of biochemistry samples sent through the post as whole blood arrive at their destination haemolysed, often so badly that no tests can be carried out. It is therefore essential for all practices, not just those with their own laboratories, to equip themselves with a centrifuge for sample separation. Heparinised samples (and fluoride/oxalate samples) may be spun and the plasma separated immediately. However, clotted samples must be left for at least two hours for the clot to form before the serum can be separated. If the use of clotted samples is unavoidable, then glass tubes must be used, as plastic tubes promote haemolysis while the clot is forming. If a bucket centrifuge is used, then about 10 minutes centrifugation at 2,500—3,000 rpm will be adequate for most samples, while with a dual purpose microhaematocrit centrifuge, only 2—3 minutes is necessary due to the higher speed. The use of plastic beads of jelly ('Serasieve', Hughes & Hughes) aids separation, and the jelly will actually allow the plasma to be poured off, thus avoiding the need for a pasteur pipette. It is important that the plasma be transferred to another tube as prolonged contact with the cells, even after centrifugation, will lead to changes in plasma composition.

Storage and Preservation

Plasma samples should be kept in the fridge ($+4^{\circ}C$), and any which are to be kept for more than two or three days should be frozen ($-20^{\circ}C$). However, repeated freezing and thawing should be avoided as this can cause deterioration of some enzymes.

Deterioration

Haemolysis is the main cause of deterioration to biochemistry samples, and may occur at sampling due to faulty technique or later due to delay in plasma or serum separation. If samples are centrifuged soon after collection, any haemolysis must be an actual sampling problem (except in rare cases of acute haemolytic disease) and this can be investigated and corrected. Delay in centrifugation will cause originally perfectly good samples to become haemolysed and unusable, and should be avoided at all costs. Exposure to heat and light, for example, on the dashboard of a car, will rapidly induce haemolysis. Time itself will cause deterioration in most enzymes and a few other substances such as creatinine, and exposure to light will cause bilirubin to decompose. These effects may be minimised by keeping samples refrigerated or frozen, in the dark.

Transport of samples is dealt with on page 149. Appendix 2.

LABORATORY METHODS

SIMPLE TESTS

Simple dipstix-type tests are available which measure urea and glucose in whole blood and which require no laboratory equipment.

Azostix (Ames) give a qualitative estimation of urea up to about 20 mmol/l in four stages. They are useful as a quick screen but, as they cannot distinguish between the moderately and the grossly elevated, raised results must be backed up by an accurate analysis before any drastic action is taken.

Dextrostix (Ames) give a semi-quantitive estimation of glucose up to about 14 mmol/l in seven stages. They have now been superseded by the two following products which are more accurate and have a wider useful range.

B-M test glycaemie (BCL) measure glucose up to 44 mmol/l in eight stages. They utilise double colour blocks which require a little practice to read accurately.

Glucostix (Ames) is a recent addition to the market which is essentially identical to the B-M test glycaemie.

General Guidelines

These products are all accompanied by detailed instructions (they are intended, in fact, for self-testing by human patients) and it is unnecessary to repeat these here. There are, however, a few general points to be borne in mind.

1. Store strips at **room temperature**, away from high humidity and in their original container.

2. Remove only the **strip to be used and do not** return unused strips to the bottle.

3. Replace cap firmly immediately after removing strip.

4. Do not touch the reagent pad or let it touch other objects.

5. Always follow the manufacturer's instructions carefully and in full.

6. Cover the **whole of the reagent pad with a** liberal drop of blood and ensure that this goes on the right side of the strip.

7. Throw out all strips past their expiry date (where this date depends on the date when the bottle was first opened, ensure that this is recorded).

8. Never transfer strips from one bottle to another.

PHOTOMETER METHODS

Beyond these simple tests the backbone of biochemical analysis is the photometer, and it is the choice of this instrument which will have the most impact on the ease and scope of operations in the area. The variety of instruments available is wide, almost bewilderingly so, but the system concepts can be divided into two basic groups:— open and closed systems.

Open Systems

In this system a basic filter photometer is used with reagents purchased from any commercial source, quite often the same type of reagent kits used by larger clinical analysers. The main advantage is that virtually any routine test can (theoretically) be run on these instruments. However, the non-standardised nature of the reagent pack means that the amount of physical manipulation (pipetting, mixing, diluting, timing, reading, calculating, etc.) involved between sample and the result is often considerable. This is not only time consuming and labour intensive, it allows a large number of opportunities for gross operator error, which can be a serious disadvantage to practices relying on non-technical staff (i.e. nurses and vets) to perform the tests. Another point of caution is that the bulk reagent packs, which often appear very cheap on a per-test basis, may not be quite so cheap when wastage due to time expiry is taken into account. When choosing a photometer as the basis of an open system, it is prudent to choose one with as many of the following features as possible in order to cut down the number of operator steps and hence reduce the chances of operator error and simplify staff training.

1. Peltier cell to control cuvette temperature.

2. Flow-through cuvette.

3. Automatic filter selection.

4. Automatic zeroing.

5. Readout in concentration (rather than absorbance) units.

6. Automatic calculation of reaction rates in kinetic tests.

7. Intelligent microprocessor control to allow standard curves to be stored in memory.

As the necessity to bring a water bath up to temperature can seriously hamper out-of-hours use, it is important to include a dry heating block for test incubation as this may be left on permanently with little maintenance required.

Three open systems, each backed by a range of test kits, are currently (or have recently been) marketed specifically to veterinary surgeons.

The BCL 4010 system. This incorporates a basic photometer with few of the features listed above. Some kits have been designed specifically for the machine while others are simply those sold for general use, and so ease of operation, comprehensibility of instructions and availability of small reagent packs (to cut down wastage in kits with a short shelf-life) is variable.

The Vitalab 21 system (VetLab). This is based around a more sophisticated photometer with most of the features listed above. The system is marketed by a veterinary company (Vetlab Supplies) and is designed with the veterinary surgeon specifically in mind. Although this is probably the most successful attempt to structure an open system for veterinary use, it does not approach the closed systems so far as simplicity of operation is concerned.

The Ames Quick-Lab system (development of the Compur M2000S system). Again, the photometer involved is sophisticated — but in this case perhaps too sophisticated, as it incorporates such things as human reference ranges to which it draws attention by a display of flashing lights when a result falls outside these ranges; this could soon become very irritating in a veterinary practice. Additional disadvantages are that many of the reagents appear to be available only in uneconomically large volumes and that methods are cumbersome.

Closed Systems

In a closed system, the measuring instrument, its programming and the reagent kits are designed together, with simplicity of operation the prime objective. The main advantages for the lay operator are improved accessibility, reduced time taken for results to be available, reduced staff training requirements and, most importantly, a reduction in opportunities for operator error. The disadvantages are that the machines are tied, usually irrevocably, to their own reagent kits. These tend to be expensive compared to the bulk reagents offered with open systems and may limit the test choice available. Closed systems are, however, excellent choices as a first foray into lab work by a practice with little or no prior experience. Their user-friendliness ensures maximum utilisation, and if all goes well, then advancement to an open system may be considered after a few years. It is usually dangerous to go from complete reliance on an outside lab to complete do-it-yourself in one fell swoop, and attempts to do this can leave expensive equipment under-utilised because of lack of expertise.

Five closed systems are, or have been, available to the veterinary market. Two of these are traditional transmission/absorbance photometers while the other three are reflectance photometers, which operate in a quite novel way, measuring changes in light reflected off a wet, solid-state reagent pad.

The Bio-dynamics (BCL) Unimeter system. This older, single wavelength photometer is no longer available but is still quite widely used. There is an extensive but expensive range of kits supplied with all necessities such as pipette tips. Instructions are extremely comprehensive, almost infuriatingly so, and the instrument itself is simple to use. However, many of the methods are multi-stage and time consuming.

The Sclavo Uni-fast system (Trio diagnostics). This is based on a sophisticated photometer with all the features listed on page 26, linked to a set of kits which is cleverly designed so that operator steps are both minimised and standardised for all methods. The range of tests available is usefully wide and the system is probably as user-friendly as it is possible to get while remaining with a transmission/absorbance instrument. It has the additional advantage of not being irrevocably tied to its custom-made kits, being usable as an open system if required — this would allow extra tests to be added to the menu (though at the cost of greater operator labour).

The Ames Seralyser. This is the oldest of the reflectance meters and is quite widely used. It has about ten tests of veterinary importance, it is quite simple to use, the reagents are the cheapest of all closed systems and its reading time is very fast (30 seconds to 4 minutes). Plasma samples require to be diluted before use, but this is, in some ways, an advantage as it eliminates the inter-species differences in plasma viscosity which can be a problem with veterinary samples on these instruments.

The Kodak Ektachem. This is the largest and most expensive of all the systems discussed and, for a reflectance meter, it has an extremely wide range of tests available. It is reasonably simple to operate. Unfortunately, it appears that its use of neat plasma results in definite problems in a number of tests when non-human samples are used and the manufacturer's own data reveal much poorer correlation with reference methods in animal species.

The BCL Reflotron. This reflectance meter is currently the ultimate in ease of operation and user friendliness. It requires no dilution and no calibration and is fast in operation (2−5 minutes). It is even possible to run whole blood on this machine, eliminating the need for centrifugation of samples, although considering that the plasma separation system built into the reagent strips is not so efficient with small (animal) erythrocytes as it is with the larger human cells, it is probably prudent to forego this luxury. There are about nine tests of veterinary importance − a tenth, γGT, appears not to work on non-human samples.

General Operational Points

As the actual test protocol is dependent on the system chosen and varies from test to test in the open systems, it is impossible to give detailed step-by-step instructions for the actual performing of biochemical tests. However, a few general points may be of use.

Automatic pipettes are quicker and easier to use than glass pipettes, are more accurate at small volumes, avoid the requirement for suction by mouth and eliminate tedious washing of glassware. However, operators must become familiar with their operation.

1. Always use the correct size of tip for each pipette.

2. Release the plunger slowly, avoiding splashing or bubbles.

3. Ensure that the fluid does **not** touch the end of the pipette or become sucked into it. This is especially important when using the reverse pipette method, where more than the required volume of fluid is aspirated, leaving a residue in the tip after dispensing − a more accurate method for slightly viscous fluids.

4. Always wipe the outside of the tip before dispensing − but avoid blotting the end.

5. Discard the used tip before proceeding to pipette a different fluid.

The purchase of two variable volume pipettes (20−200 μl and 200−1000 μl) is probably the most economical way of equipping an open system, although it will take longer to set the required volume than to select the appropriate size from a rack of fixed volume-pipettes. Closed systems will have their pipettes supplied and the manufacturer's instructions should be followed carefully. The pipette supplied with the Unimeter system is of unusual design, dispensing one of two volumes (13 μl or 97.5 μl) depending on which stop is used, and requires particular care. It is a wash-out pipette, not a delivery-volume; the exact volume is in the tip and must be washed out with solvent. This means that it cannot be used to pipette into a dry tube, and that each tip cannot be used more than once, even to pipette the same fluid.

Transmission/absorbance photometry is the traditional 'wet chemistry' method and both open and closed systems require some pipetting and mixing. Mixing of the reaction mixture is important and should be done with a flick of the wrist without covering or spilling − the use of parafilm is extremely time-consuming. In most systems it is advisable to set (or re-set) the blank immediately before reading the sample. Where individual cuvettes are in use these should be carefully wiped before placing in the instrument to clear the light path and, of course, cuvettes must never be labelled! Where filters must be changed by hand, care must be taken to avoid fingermarks or dust on the filter. Many photometers require a warm-up period after switching on and it may be just as convenient to keep them on permanently.

Endpoint methods are simple procedures where one measurement is taken after a reaction is complete and the absorbance is proportional to the concentration of the analyte, the constant being derived from the standard curve. It is important to allow the correct incubation period − too short and the colour will not be fully developed, too long and it may begin to fade. When a value is obtained which is higher than the limit of sensitivity of the assay, the test **must** be repeated using either an appropriate dilution of the sample or a smaller volume, and the result multiplied. With photometers which can store standard curves, it is important to recalibrate these curves as recommended by the manufacturers or when quality control results (see below) indicate that this is necessary.

Kinetic methods are generally used to measure enzymes and require a number of measurements to be taken to establish the rate at which a reaction is proceeding. Many photometers will do this automatically and do not require to be sat over with a stopwatch and a pencil and paper. A lag phase is always allowed in kinetic methods to allow the reaction to get started and on to its linear phase. However, in some samples with very high enzyme activity, the whole reaction may have gone to its endpoint during the lag period before the first reading is taken. This can be identified by the fact that this first reading — the **initial absorbance** — is much higher than it ought to be (or lower if the reaction is a descending one), and the reaction rate is non-linear or virtually zero. Such samples must be diluted and re-run and it is important to be alert to this phenomenon — known as **'substrate exhaustion'** — to avoid reporting an extremely pathological enzyme value as normal.

Reflectance photometry is confined to closed systems and little understanding of theory is required. The basic endpoint and kinetic methods are much the same in principle but, in general, the machines are designed to do most of the thinking. Careful pipetting is again important, and it is usually necessary to practise pipetting with a very steady hand as the tip must not touch the reagent pad. In most systems, reasonably swift, practised movement is essential, as once the sample is pipetted, the subsequent closing and startup of the machine must not be delayed too long. When samples must be diluted, great care should be taken. Even in systems which normally use neat plasma, the basic essentials for sample dilution (pipettes, tips, distilled water) must be to hand to cope with over-range samples.

QUALITY ASSURANCE

In its fullest sense, this means that good samples, promptly delivered to the laboratory, are analysed rapidly by a **precise, accurate** method. The results are then matched to the correct patient and reported to the appropriate clinician. Thus, the entire laboratory procedure must be scrutinised to ensure that each of these stages is organised for optimum efficiency and that there are no procedural 'black holes' into which samples or results can vanish without trace. General logistics, paperwork design, staff training, supervision, troubleshooting, ordering of supplies, waste disposal and cleaning are all involved here. It is impossible to go into detail on every aspect, but the appreciation of **precision** and **accuracy** of methods must be considered further.

Quality Control

This is the measure of the precision of an assay, and in large laboratories involved the inclusion in every batch of one (or often two) samples with known results. These are quite separate from any calibrators or standards and are not used to calculate standard curves. Limits of acceptability are pre-set and, if quality control results fall outside these limits, then the entire assay run is discarded and repeated. Cumulative quality control results provide a measure of the precision of the assay, that is the ability to get the same results repeatably, from the **coefficient of variation** (cv).

$$CV = \frac{\text{Standard deviation (SD)}}{\bar{\chi} \text{ or mean}} \times 100 \, (\%)$$

A CV of under 5% is usually considered desirable for simple tests.

In a smaller practice laboratory where tests are run singly, this procedure cannot be followed exactly — however, a reasonably designed compromise is essential. The running of one (or preferably two) quality control samples for each test at the start of each week, is probably acceptable. If the results are recorded on a graph as shown in Figure 2.2., it provides early warning of developing problems before the situation is bad enough to necessitate scrapping all results.

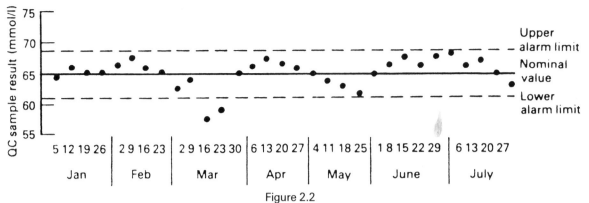

Figure 2.2

Example QC results recorded graphically, Method is 'out of control' if (a) two consecutive 'outlier' values occur, e.g. in March, (b) seven consecutive falling (or rising) values occur, e.g. in April/May, or (c) seven consecutive results above (or below) the nominal value occur, e.g. in June/July. If possible, it is better to derive your own nominal values and alarm limits for each batch of QC serum, for your own methods. Assay the QC sample every day for 10 days; nominal value is the mean and the alarm limits the $\pm$ 3SD values. Mean should be within manufacturers' specified tolerances and CV should be reasonable for the method.

The purchase of commercially prepared quality control sera is the most satisfactory approach and most preparations will give some indication of the approximate nominal values and range for most constituents. However, it is best to use equine or bovine sera (not human) to avoid risk of infections such as hepatitis or HIV.

Quality Assessment

This is the measure of the accuracy of an assay and, in large laboratories, involves the reception from an outside source of samples whose results are unknown to the laboratory staff. These are analysed as if they were patient samples and results reported to the organiser. Performance is then graded and scored in relation to other participating laboratories, with the concensus mean from all labs taken as the 'correct' result. Accuracy in this context involves getting as close as possible to this 'correct' answer.

In a smaller practice laboratory, membership of an organised scheme is not usually practical. However, it can be instructive for the supervisor either to split a patient sample and send the other half to a reliable outside laboratory (which, one hopes, will belong to a national scheme itself), or to slip in an extra quality control sample, preferably of a different batch from that in routine use, in the guise of a fictitous patient. While staff should ideally not know that a particular sample is a quality assessment specimen, it is important that results, good or bad, be discussed with them afterwards.

INTERPRETATION OF RESULTS

GENERAL CONSIDERATIONS

Many lists of 'reference values' for biochemical constituents may be found in various publications, but the fact that they seldom agree exactly, demonstrates the artificiality of adopting too rigid an approach. The fact is that on either side of 'normal' for any constituent there is a grey area in which results may or may not be abnormal (see Figure 2.3), and the decision as to the clinical relevance of such results will rest on how they fit in with other clinical and laboratory findings. Consequently, only approximate reference values are given here. The situation regarding enzymes is even less clear-cut, as the distribution of 'normal' values is generally asymmetrical, with a long tail leading into quite high figures (see Figure 2.4). This makes it very difficult to give clear upper reference limits for enzyme activities. This fact, combined with the problem of different analytical methods and temperatures giving numerically different results even when expressed as 'international units', is the reason for omitting reference values for enzymes from this chapter.

The other major consideration is that of the magnitude of the abnormality. While it is true that a grossly elevated plasma urea concentration is almost certainly indicative of renal insufficiency and a grossly elevated plasma glucose concentration probably diagnostic of diabetes mellitus, slight to moderate departures from normal may be caused by quite unrelated factors. For example, poor circulation secondary to dehydration or cardiac failure may cause a moderate elevation in urea, while extreme excitement may cause moderate hyperglycaemia. It is therefore important to appreciate the exact implications of each result and not to jump to the most obvious conclusion by reflex action.

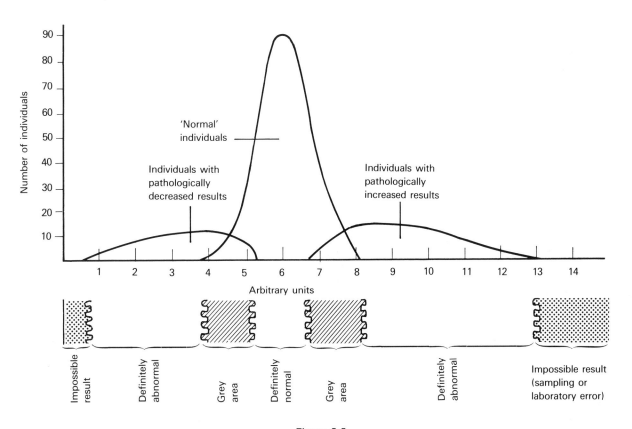

Figure 2.3
Schematic representation of the distribution of results for a figurative laboratory test
showing overlaps of 'normal' and pathological ranges.

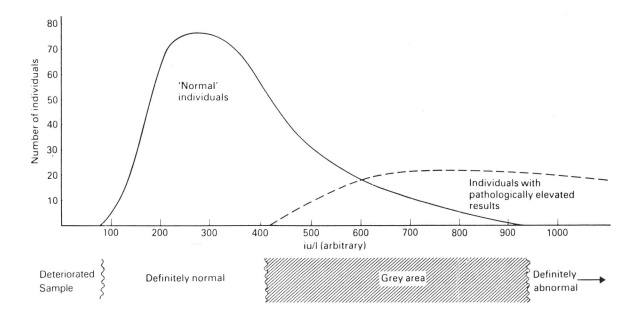

Figure 2.4
Schematic representation of the distribution of results for a figurative plasma enzyme assay,
showing how the skewed distribution of 'normal' results leads to a very wide 'grey' area.

THE PLASMA PROTEINS

Normal total plasma protein concentration is around 55—75 g/l in dogs and 60—80 g/l in cats. Of this, about 25—35 g/l is albumin and the remaining 25—40 g/l 'globulins'.

Raised total protein levels may be due to dehydration, in which case both albumin and globulins will be increased in proportion, or to an increase in one or more of the globulin fractions alone, in which case the albumin concentration will be normal or low. This latter situation is often seen as a non-specific finding in sick cats and in chronic and immune mediated diseases in all species. Cirrhosis of the liver, chronic sub-acute bacterial infections and auto-immune disease are frequently involved, and in particular FIP is often associated with a very marked hypergammaglobulinaemia together with slight hypoalbuminaemia. Identification of the particular globulin fraction involved, either by electrophoresis or by specific assay of the so-called 'acute phase proteins' (including C-reactive protein, hapotglobin and fibrinogen) which are typical of acute inflammatory disease, can often be useful. Electrophoresis will also pick out the rare cases of *paraproteinaemia,* where a malignant myeloma causes the very sharp monoclonal spike of a single immunoglobulin to appear on the trace.

Slightly depressed total protein concentrations may be a general consequence of debility, but significantly low concentrations, in particular where there is hypoalbuminaemia, are usually due either to pathological loss of protein or to decreased protein synthesis. The possible routes of protein loss include the kidney (protein-losing nephropathy), the gut (protein-losing enteropathy), haemorrhage and severe burns. Decrease protein synthesis may be due to dietary protein deficiency (uncommon in small animals), malabsorption (often accompanying protein-losing enteropathy) and liver failure. A moderate hypoalbuminaemia is sometimes seen in dogs with severe polyarthritis. It is useful to note that in intestinal protein loss both albumin and globulins are usually low, while in liver failure and protein-losing nephropathy globulins are usually normal or even raised.

THE ELECTROLYTES

The subject of electrolyte disturbances is a complex one and only a few general points can be made here. The vast majority of sodium problems are primarily fluid problems, and to a certain extent this is true of potassium also. It is important that both electrolytes should be monitored wherever possible in patients receiving fluid therapy. Other electrolytes (chloride, bicarbonate) are less frequently used in small animal practice.

Sodium

Normal plasma sodium concentration is about 140—155 mmol/l. Hypernatraemia is usually associated with loss of a low-sodium fluid, especially in vomiting, and when restricted water intake is preventing normal sodium excretion. Hyponatraemia occurs when there is a loss of a high-sodium fluid, for example when there is a failure of renal concentrating ability, or when a loss of any sodium-containing fluid is replaced by a very low-sodium fluid (for example by drinking water or I/V dextrose saline). Addison's disease is also associated with severe hyponatraemia in many cases.

Potassium

Normal plasma potassium concentration is about 4.0—5.5 mmol/l. Hyperkalaemia may be seen in cases of acute renal failure, but the first condition which should probably be considered when this finding is encountered is Addison's disease, and a Na/K ratio of less than 27:1 is a strong pointer to this diagnosis. However, note that an artificially high potassium will be seen in haemolysed samples and samples in which the plasma of serum has not been separated reasonably promptly after collection (8 hours is probably the limit). Hypokalaemia is most commonly due to loss of a high-potassium fluid, i.e. diarrhoea and/orvomiting, and cases of chronic renal failure are often hyperkalaemic due to vomiting. It is also seen frequently in patients on prolonged fluid therapy with potassium-free fluids — a classic cause of the 'downer dog' — and on prolonged frusemide therapy (however, note that some other diuretics, e.g. spironolactone, actually cause potassium retention).

THE MINERALS

Calcium

Normal plasma calcium concentration is about 2.0—3.0 mmol/l. Hypercalcaemia is a rare clinical finding. Mild hypercalcaemia may be seen in dehydrated animals or as an artefact of drip-bleeding, but genuine hypercalcaemia is only caused by primary hyperparathyroidism of some type. Primary pseudohyperparathyroidism is the usual diagnosis, generally secondary to a lymphosarcoma, usually a mediastinal one, but parathyroid adenoma is occasionally encountered. Hypocalcaemia is comparatively common, seen in eclampsia and in a proportion of cases of acute pancreatitis, and a mild and asymptomatic hypocalcaemia is often associated with hypoalbuminaemia and with chronic renal failure.

Phosphate

Normal plasma phosphate concentration is about 0.8—2.5 mmol/l. Hyperphosphataemia is the more pronounced mineral abnormality seen in chronic renal failure (due to secondary renal hyperparathyroidism) and this is the usual reason (other than haemolysis) for this finding. In growing pups, especially in large breeds, too low a dietary Ca/PO_4 ratio can also lead to hyperphosphataemia and sometimes to slight hypocalcaemia. Hypophosphataemia is an uncommon clinical finding in small animals.

VITAMIN ANALYSIS

The vitamins usually investigated in canine practice are vitamin B_{12} and folic acid. Both are useful in the differential diagnosis of intestinal malabsorption in dogs, but their relevance to the cat is uncertain and appears not to have been investigated. Normal plasma B_{12} concentration is above 200 pg/ml, and normal plasma folate concentration is 3—13 ng/ml. Low plasma B_{12} levels are associated with distal small intestinal disease, with bacterial overgrowth of the intestine and with absence of normal gastric secretion. High folate levels are also sometimes seen in cases of bacterial overgrowth, while low folate concentration is indicative of proximal small intestinal disease.

THE NITROGENOUS SUBSTANCES

Urea

Normal plasma urea concentration is about 2—8 mmol/l in dogs and up to about 15 mmol/l in cats. Note that the term BUN refers specifically to a particular unit of measurement, now long outdated, and its use in the context of SI units is incorrect.

Slightly raised plasma urea concentrations may be due to certain dietary or metabolic factors, especially where excess protein is being broken down, and is also seen in cases of chronic intestinal haemorrhage. Moderately raised concentrations (up to about 20—30 mmol/l) may well be due to a degree of renal dysfunction, but circulatory failure should also be considered especially if creatinine concentration is normal or only slightly raised. Conditions which may lead to this degree of circulatory failure are severe dehydration, advanced cardiac failure, and Addison's disease (especially Addisonian crisis). Once plasma urea concentration is over about 35 mmol/l, primary renal or post-renal problems are almost certainly involved. Renal failure (acute or chronic) is the most usual cause. However, the possibilities of urethral obstruction or ruptured bladder should not be overlooked.

Low plasma urea concentrations are an infrequent occurrence, and several possibilities must be considered:

1.   Metabolic idiosyncracy of normal animal.
2.   Dietary protein insufficiency — usually seen as a consequence of anorexia in small animals.
3.   Inborn error of the urea cycle (congenital condition which presents in the young animal).
4.   Congenital portocaval shunt (also young animals).
5.   Severe liver disease often with an acquired portocaval shunt.

In these last three conditions the low urea will be accompanied by hyperammonaemia (see below).

Creatinine

Normal plasma creatinine concentration is under about 120 μmol/l in dogs and under about 180 μmol/l in cats.

Raised plasma creatinine concentration is a more specific indicator of renal or post-renal problems than urea as it is less affected by pre-renal conditions (dietary or circulatory). Creatinine levels of up to about 200 μmol/l may accompany severe circulatory problems (in which case the urea will be well over 20 mmol/l), but, above this figure, renal (or post-renal) problems are a virtual certainty. The practice of measuring both urea and creatinine has many advantages, with the urea offering a wider metabolic view and the creatinine helping to identify the cause of any abnormality.

Ammonia

Normal plasma ammonia concentration is under about 60 μmol/l in most species.

Hyperammonaemia (values above 100 μmol/l) is a feature of three specific conditions: inborn error of the urea cycle, congenital porto-caval shunt, and end-stage liver failure. In the majority of cases, plasma urea concentration is also low. End-stage liver is seldom difficult to diagnose on other biochemical tests, and it is the only one of these conditions which can affect the older animal. Differentiation of the two congenital conditions can be tricky, however. As a guide, porto-caval shunt cases usually show evidence of dysfunction of other aspects of liver metabolism (hypoalbuminaemia and raised liver enzymes for example) while inborn error cases do not, but often a portal angiogram is the only way to reach a positive diagnosis. Note that samples for ammonia estimation must be kept on ice and processed and analysed within a very short time of collection — this completely rules out posting samples to a distant laboratory.

CARBOHYDRATE METABOLISM

Glucose

Normal fasting plasma glucose concentration is about 4—6 mmol/l in all monogastric species.

Slight hyperglycaemia (up to about 7 mmol/l) is seen in the hours following a meal, as a result of moderate stress or excitement, and in a proportion of cases of Cushing's syndrome. Slightly more marked hyperglycaemia (up to about 15 mmol/l) may occur as a result of extreme excitement, or the over-enthusiastic administration of glucose-containing I/V fluids. Cases of diabetes mellitus may show plasma glucose concentrations of anything from 8 mmol/l (mild cases) to as much as 60 mmol/l.

Hypoglycaemia is an unusual cause of fainting and other nervous signs, in dogs more often than in cats. It is important to try to sample as soon after a fit as possible, as a normal result may well be obtained at other times. Possible causes include overdosage of therapeutic insulin, insulinoma (malignancy of the islet cells of the pancreas), non-malignant islet-cell hyperplasia (uncommon) and an 'idiopathic' hypoglycaemia seen in toy breeds of dog. A very slight hypoglycaemia (3—4 mmol/l) is often seen in Addison's disease. Note that samples taken into a tube which does not contain fluoride will appear hypoglycaemic unless processed and analysed very soon after collection.

Glycosylated Haemoglobin

This test is used in human medicine as a part of diabetic monitoring and is beginning to attract some interest in veterinary medicine also. The percentage of haemoglobin molecules which are glycosylated is a function of the mean plasma glucose concentration over the preceding 3—4 months — in normal animals about 5—10%. Thus, this measurement can provide some information about the degree of control achieved over this period in a diabetic patient. Note, however, that the test is an adjunct to, not a substitute for, regular blood (and urine) monitoring. It must also be appreciated that it is not useful during initial diagnosis or stabilisation.

'Ketone Bodies'

The ketone most usually measured nowadays is ß-hydroxybutyrate, and normal plasma concentration of this is under 1 mmol/l (often undetectable). In monogastrics the only type of ketosis usually encountered is diabetic ketoacidoses. Such animals are grossly hyperglycaemic and frequently in, or about to enter, a diabetic coma. While measurement of plasma ß-hydroxybutyrate will certainly demonstrate the ketosis, checking a urine sample with a dipstick with a ketone patch is equally satisfactory and usually much quicker. Close attention to plasma potassium levels is, however, very important when treating these patients. Ketosis due to starvation is seldom encountered in monogastric animals.

BILIRUBIN AND FAT METABOLISM

Bilirubin

Normal plasma concentration is under about 5 μmol/l in small animals, but concentrations under 10 μmol/l are fairly unremarkable. Note that in small animals, where the plasma is normally colourless, measurement of bilirubin is unnecessary unless there is a yellow colour present in the plasma. Conversely, where a plasma sample is seen to be yellow, bilirubin should always be investigated.

There are three specific causes of raised plasma bilirubin levels:

1. Intravascular haemolysis. Jaundice due to haemolytic disease is usually fairly mild, about 10—20 μmol/l, and in chronic haemolytic conditions (particularly autoimmune haemolytic anaemia) it may be absent. These patients will be anaemic, and the red cell picture will be regenerative (again with the exception of many autoimmune haemolytic anaemia cases). Almost all the bilirubin will be unconjugated.

2. Liver failure. There are two basic categories of liver disease in which jaundice is a feature — acute hepatitis, where the jaundice often disappears just as suddenly as it came, and in which it is not necessarily a poor prognostic sign, and end-stage liver failure, where the gradual onset of jaundice is often a terminal feature. Prolonged severe hyperbilirubinaemia, sometimes with normal liver enzymes, is often indicative of hepatic neoplasia. Differentiation of conjugated/unconjugated bilirubin may be unrewarding.

3. Biliary obstruction, either intra- or extra-hepatic. Again, tumours are a common cause. Plasma bilirubin can be very high in such cases, even up to 500 μmol/l, and in the early stages most of it is conjugated. Later, 'damming-back' will increase the unconjugated proportion. Plasma alkaline phosphatase activity will also be very high in these cases and, where the obstruction is complete, the faeces are usually pale.

Bile Acids

Normal plasma total bile acid concentration is under about 15 μmol/l.

This test has now generally replaced the BSP clearance test as a measure of hepatic anion transport due to both ease of performance and better sensitivity. However, the test is generally irrelevant if obvious jaundice is present (as bile acid levels will certainly be high also). It is of value in cases of genuine doubt as to whether a mild jaundice is haemolytic or hepatic. Bile acid measurements are most useful as a second line of investigation where differential diagnosis of hypoalbuminaemia is the problem, or where liver enzymes have been found to be elevated over a prolonged period and information on the state of liver function is therefore required. Note that bile acids, like bilirubin, also rise in cases of acute hepatitis and in this circumstance do not necessarily indicate a poor prognosis.

Cholesterol

Normal plasma cholesterol concentration is under about 7.5 mmol/l in dogs and under about 5 mmol/l in cats.

Slight hypercholesterolaemia is seen after a recent fatty meal, and so it is important to obtain a true fasting sample for this test. Moderately raised cholesterol concentrations are seen in hepatobiliary disease, nephrotic syndrome and diabetes mellitus, but the test is not really of diagnostic importance in these conditions. The majority of cases of Cushing's syndrome exhibit a moderate hypercholesterolaemia, around 10—12 mmol/l, but the most spectacularly increased cholesterol levels are caused by hypothyroidism. Concentrations can rise as high as 50 mmol/l, and this sort of finding is virtually pathognomonic for this condition (note, however, that about one-third of hypothyroid cases have normal plasma cholesterol concentrations).

Unusually low plasma cholesterol concentrations are sometimes seen in cases of hyperthyroidism, but the test is of little diagnostic use in this context.

ENZYMES

Enzymes are present in the plasma more or less by accident. When a cell dies or is badly damaged its contents, including enzyme molecules, leak out into the interstitial fluid and thence to the plasma. As cells of different tissues contain different enzymes, it is possible by this means to detect damage to particular organs. (Note, however, that **damage** to an organ does not necessarily imply failure of that organ — enzymes seldom give any information about organ **function**). One enzyme is seldom totally specific for one particular tissue, but it is usually possible to localise the damage by looking at a number of different enzymes, or (more precise but involving more analytical difficulty) by investigating the isoenzymes involved — these often are specific for a particular tissue.

Creatine kinase (CK) is virtually specific for striated muscle. There are also cardiac muscle and brain isoenzymes but these are of little diagnostic importance in the small animal field. Note also that a slight increase in CK activity is often seen in cases of hypothyroidism, due to a reduction in excretion.

Lactate dehydrogenase (LDH) has five isoenzymes and is associated with both skeletal and cardiac muscle, liver, kidney, lung and erythrocytes. Due to its wide distribution, total LDH levels are often of little use unless isoenzyme estimation is also available.

Aspartate aminotransferase (AST, formerly GOT) is associated with both muscle (striated and cardiac) and liver. Due to the better specificity of ALT for liver in small animals, AST is used almost exclusively to investigate muscle damage in these species.

Alanine aminotransferase (ALT, formerly GPT) is also associated with both muscle and liver, but in small animals the vast majority of this enzyme is hepatic in origin. It is generally a good indicator of hepatocellular damage in these species, though small, non-specific increases are sometimes seen.

Gamma glutamyl transferase (αGT or GGT) tends to parallel ALT activity in cases of hepatocellular damage in dogs, but with rather less sensitivity. It seldom provides any useful information over and above that provided by ALT. In cats, plasma αGT activity is extremely low (frequently undetectable) and increases are uncommon.

Alkaline phosphatase (ALP) has several isoenzymes, notably bone (osteoblasts), liver and intestinal wall, plus a biliary isoenzyme which is produced during biliary stasis and a steroid-induced isoenzyme which also originates from the liver. There is also a high activity in the skin. The test is particularly useful in cases when fatty infiltration of the liver has occurred e.g. diabetes mellitus.

α-**Amylase (AMS)** is present in the pancreas of dogs, and plasma activity increases very markedly in cases of acute pancreatitis. Smaller non-specific increases may occur in other acute abdominal conditions and also in chronic renal failure, due to a reduction in excretion.

Lipase is also a pancreatic enzyme. Plasma levels increase more slowly at the beginning of an attack of acute pancreatitis, compared to amylase, and remain elevated for longer.

Immunoreactive trypsin (IRT or TLI) is a molecule, similar to trypsin but not proteolytically active, which is present in the plasma. Again, its source is the pancreas. While it also increases in acute pancreatitis, its clinical usefulness is in the diagnosis of exocrine pancreatic insufficiency in dogs where it is, in fact, an organ function test. Where there is aplasia or atrophy of the pancreas, plasma levels **decline** appreciably. Note that total amylase or lipase activities are not useful tests in this context.

HORMONES

Sex Hormones

The sex hormones most commonly measured in small animal practice are oestradiol, progesterone and testosterone. This type of investigation may be useful in identifying the reasons for a supposedly neutered animal continuing to exhibit sexual behaviour. The use of hormonal analyses in cases of infertility is limited on economic grounds as repeated measurements are usually necessary to obtain any useful information, and there appears to be no benefit in this type of measurement in cases of skin disease.

Metabolic Hormones

Cortisol is elevated in a single resting sample in only a small proportion of cases of Cushing's disease and an ACTH stimulation test (or dexamethasone screening, see below) is really necessary to make a definite diagnosis. A single low cortisol reading may be rather more helpful in diagnosing Addison's disease, if other relevant signs are present, but again an ACTH stimulation test is best carried out.

Thyroxine (T_4) is useful in investigating both hypothroidism and hyperthyroidism. A single sample is usually sufficient to diagnose hyperthyroidism, with T_4 values over 70 nmol/l being suspicious and those over 100 nmol/l virtually conclusive. The interpretation of low values is less clear cut, however. Results of under 10 nmol/l are a generally good indication of hypothyroidism, especially when other indications are present, but similar T_4 levels can occur in other conditions, notably Cushing's syndrome, and so complete reliance on one test is unwise. Values of 10—20 nmol/l are possibly indicative of hypothyroidism, but inconclusive, while at levels over 20 nmol/l hypothyroidism is unlikely, becoming less likely with increasing T_4 levels. Clarification of the situation can be provided by measuring free (unbound) T_4 levels, and/or by carrying out a TRH stimulation test.

Tri-iodothyronine (T_3) is probably a secondary test nowadays, but it does provide additional useful information particularly where thyroid carcinoma is suspected. The older criterion for hypothyroidism — two of the three tests, T_4, T_3 and cholesterol being abnormal — is still occasionally useful also.

Insulin estimation is seldom necessary in the diagnosis of diabetes mellitus, but it may be required in the investigation of cases which are secondary to the presence of an insulin antagonist. This insulin-resistant form of the disease (sometimes occurring in animals with Cushing's syndrome, among other things) is characterised by a normal or raised plasma insulin level (over about 20 mU/l) in the presence of persistent hyperglycaemia. Insulin measurement is also vital for the diagnosis of insulinoma, when high levels (usually over 80 mU/l) are seen in the presence of hypoglycaemia.

DYNAMIC TESTING

In many situations much more information may be gained by looking at changes in plasma levels of a constituent following the administration of a stimulant or a depressant, than can be gained by looking only at random or resting levels. As a rather large number of such tests have been described over the years, only those most commonly used in small animal medicine are discussed here.

Bromosulphthalein (BSP) Clearance Test

This test of hepatic function (specifically hepatic anion transport) is falling out of use due to the increase in popularity of bile acid measurements, but may be briefly described. BSP is injected intravenously at a dose rate of 5 mg/kg and its rate of decay in the plasma followed. Protocols which involve the taking of only one sample at 30 min post injection may be somewhat suspect as they rely on an estimation of blood volume as a proportion of body weight, which may not be as expected in ascitic or obese patients. Three samples (10, 20 and 30 min) are preferable, and in this way the half-life can be calculated by plotting the results on semilog paper. Normal BSP half-life is around 4—6 min, and values of over 10 min are clinically significant. Drawbacks to this test are that BSP is not stable in blood and so postal samples are unsuitable, and adverse reactions to the BSP have been reported in human patients.

Glucose Tolerance Test (GTT)

The oral glucose tolerance test is more commonly used in veterinary practice; the intravenous test is rarely required. Even so, a full-blown (5-sample) GTT is seldom necessary, with the simplified 'two hour post glucose plasma glucose level' test being preferable for the confirmation of mild diabetes mellitus, as this protocol greatly reduces the chance of stress or excitement interfering with the results. The usual oral dose of glucose (2 g/kg) is given to the fasting animal, and a single sample collected 2 hours later. Plasma glucose of over 8 mmol/l is indicative of diabetes. In the full GTT, samples are taken at 0, 30, 60, 90 and 120 minutes. This is required to confirm a suspected renal glycosuria (simultaneous urine samples are also required), and when the test is being used to investigate intestinal malabsorption. In the former condition the GTT is normal, with glucose values never exceeding the normal renal glucose threshold (8—10 mmol/l) in spite of the glycosuria, and in the latter the curve is flat, lacking the usual peak of 7—8 mmol/l at 1 hour. (However, measurement of B_{12} and folate have generally superseded this investigation, and the similar xylose absorption test, in canine medicine).

ACTH Stimulation Test

This test is essential for the confirmation of Cushing's syndrome and is recommended for the confirmation of Addison's disease. Several protocols are described, but the following appears to give the most clear-cut interpretation.

1. Collect resting blood sample (a 9 am start is recommended but not essential).
2. Inject 0.25 mg ACTH (Synacthen, Ciba) intravenously.
3. Collect second blood sample two hours later.

In normal animals the cortisol level in the resting animal will be between 30 and 250 nmol/l, rising in the post ACTH sample to no more than 600 nmol/l. Cushing's syndrome is characterised by post ACTH cortisol values of over 1000 nmol/l (values between 600 and 1000 nmol/l are usually indicative of Cushing's but without complete certainty). A resting cortisol value of over 400 nmol/l is also virtually diagnostic, but this is only seen in a small proportion of cases. In Addison's disease a low resting cortisol (under 100 nmol/l, usually under 20 nmol/l) is seen, and there is little or no increase after ACTH injection, sometimes an actual decrease.

Dexamethasone Screening Test

This test is useful where the ACTH stimulation test has failed to give clear-cut results in suspected Cushing's syndrome. It should not be carried out on the same day as the former test.

1. Collect resting blood sample.
2. Inject 0.01 mg/kg dexamethasone intravenously.
3. Collect second blood sample 3 hours after injection.
4. Collect third blood sample 8 hours after injection.

Cushing's syndrome is characterised by a 3—hour cortisol level of more than 50% of the resting level, and an 8—hour level of over 40 nmol/l. However, some pituitary-dependent cases demonstrate normal 3—hour levels.

Dexamethasone Suppression Test

This test is designed for use in patients which have already been positively diagnosed as suffering from hyperadrenocorticism. It is intended to distinguish between pituitary dependent cases and cases of adrenal tumour, but experience has shown that it is not particularly reliable. The protocol is exactly the same as the screening test, except that the dexamethasone dose is 0.1 mg/kg. Where both the 3—hour and 8—hour cortisol values are over 50% of the resting value, an adrenal tumour is indicated. Other combinations suggest a pituitary dependent form of the condition.

TRH Stimulation Test

This test for hypothyroidism is useful in the clarification of ambiguous cases, for example where the resting T_4 level is between 10 and 20 nmol/l or where the aggregation of clinical signs and laboratory results is contradictory. It utilises thyroid releasing hormone (TRH) rather than the thyroid stimulating hormone (TSH) usually described, due to difficulties with supply of the latter substance to veterinary surgeons in the UK.

1. Collect resting blood sample.
2. Inject 200 μg TRH (Roche) intravenously.
3. Collect second sample between 4 and 6 hours later.

In normal animals the T_4 level will increase to at least 1½ times the resting level while hypothyroid animals show very little increase. However, this is only really valid where resting T_4 is low — where it is over 30 nmol/l hypothyroidism is unlikely but marked increases in T_4 may not occur post TRH. Note also that cases of secondary hypothyroidism (usually due to pituitary neoplasia) often demonstrate a normal TRH response.

ADDITIONAL INFORMATION

FURTHER READING

KERR, M. G. (1989) *Veterinary Laboratory Medicine: Clinical Biochemistry and Haematology.* Oxford: Blackwell Scientific Publications.

KANEKO, J. J. (1980) *Clinical Biochemistry of Domestic Animals,* 3rd edn. New York: Academic Press.

The figures in Chapter Two are from 'Veterinary Laboratory Medicine: Clinical Biochemistry and Haematology' by M. G. Kerr, and are reproduced by permission.

CHAPTER 3

URINE ANALYSIS

D. L. Doxey B.V.M.& S., Ph.D., M.R.C.V.S.

INTRODUCTION

Urine analysis is the one technique which almost any practice should be able to undertake. Samples can be obtained by the patient's owner in most instances and commercially available stick and tablet tests have been available at a reasonable cost for many years. In addition, the results of urine analysis have wider applications than just urinary tract dysfunction. All in all, it is a very useful ancillary diagnostic procedure which should be employed at some time by all practices; the only minor difficulties likely to arise involve those aspects of the procedure for which commercial reagents are not available or those which require microscopy. The latter requires a financial outlay but the microscope will, with care, last for many years while the former can be easily dealt with by a trained animal nurse. In short, urine analysis is the one laboratory based technique all practitioners who wish to improve their diagnostic ability should be undertaking.

SAMPLE COLLECTION

Samples may be taken during urination or by catheterisation or even by cystocentesis although I have never found the last technique useful in animals whose lower urinary tract is unobstructed. Samples may be taken by the owner or by staff within the practice premises.

Midstream free flow samples are the most representative in dogs but not always easy to obtain and somtimes the last dribble has to suffice. Whichever is obtained it is **essential** that the sample is collected into a wide necked scrupulously **clean** container. Such containers should be supplied by the practice. Do not rely on an owner to provide their own container which may look clean but contains impurities. If microbiological examinations are to be undertaken, the collection container should be sterile.

With cats in their home environment, free flow collection procedures may be impossible and in such cases hospitalisation and collection is required.

Catheterisation is necessary in cases where free flow collection is not possible. Always use sterile catheters. Bladder puncture using a syringe and sterile 20 – 24 gauge needle can be used if a catheter cannot be passed. Ensure aseptic precautions are taken.

Never collect samples by mopping up urine from the floor. Samples collected in this way will be contaminated and largely useless.

Size and storage

Sample size is not vital but try and ensure that at least 10 ml of urine is collected. Whenever possible analyse the fresh samples rapidly. When there has to be a delay of up to 24 hours, storage at 4°C in the refrigerator is acceptable although it may have some adverse effects on urine deposits. If there is to be a longer delay, use bottles already containing boric acid as a preservative (200 mg boric acid per 15 ml of urine). These are available commercially (Boricon, Medical Wire Co.). Bacteriological studies may be affected by preservatives and are best conducted on fresh urine samples.

LABORATORY METHODS

Methods for urine analysis fall into three categories:

1. Commercially available dipstick and tablet tests.
2. Tests for which no commercial kit is available.
3. Urine deposit examination.

To undertake the procedure correctly a practice laboratory should be prepared to undertake all three forms of urine analysis but often work is confined to the commercially available materials only, which is unfortunate as valuable results, such as cell content of the sample, are not obtained.

COMMERCIALLY AVAILABLE TESTS

There are two major sources of supply — Ames and Boehringer. Both firms supply a variety of tests ranging from single test sticks, for example glucose, to multiple test strips capable of evaluating 6 or 8 different values. It is very important the manufacturer's directions are followed exactly, that the tests are not used when their expiry date has passed and, most important, that the lid of the bottle is kept tightly closed when not in use. If these precautions are not followed it is quite possible to obtain test results which are at best of doubtful value and at worst completely misleading.

Users must not fall into the trap of assuming that because these tests are easy to use and give easily visible results that they are infallible. You must take just as much care with their use as with other laboratory tests if you wish to get correct results.

A variety of strip tests are available but all work on the same general principle. Each strip has a multi-layered pad attached to one end containing the various reagents required for the test. When this pad is soaked with urine, the reagents mix and a reaction occurs which culminates in a gradual colour change. The colour change is compared by eye with a chart provided by the manufacturer and a semi-quantitative or quantitative result can then be derived. Instruments to 'read' the colour changes are available which helps to avoid mistakes which can occur, for instance, with colour blindness.

The tests available from commercial sources include the following: —

pH	blood
protein	nitrite
glucose	specific gravity
ketones	leucocytes
bilirubin	antibacterial substances
urobilinogen	

OTHER CHEMICAL TESTS

A variety of tests can be undertaken for which reagents will have to be purchased individually. None of them are particularly difficult but some of the reagents, for example concentrated hydrochloric acid, have to be handled with care.

The tests can be divided into two categories:

   a. tests using different methods from the commercially available test;

   b. tests for which there is no commercial equivalent.

a. In this category are included **specific gravity** which is measured with a refractometer using a few drops of urine. The results are precise and the method rapid. The values obtained by refractometer and those obtained using stick tests may not always be the same as the methods employed use different principles. It is best to use one method or the other. Do not mix the methods if this can be avoided.

   It is, of course, possible to undertake estimations such as glucose or leucocyte detection by other methods, but these will not be considered here.

b. In this second category are two tests which are useful and should be included in a routine urine analysis whenever possible.

Bile salts — sprinkle a **little** finely divided flowers of sulphur on to the surface of the urine. If bile salts are present, surface tension is lowered and the sulphur sinks to the bottom of the test tube.

Indican

Jaffe's test: Place approximately 5 ml of urine in a test tube and add at least 2 ml of chloroform, so the chloroform is seen as a distinct clear layer at the bottom of the tube. Mix well by decanting the liquid from one test tube into another repeatedly. Add as much concentrated hydrochloric acid as urine. Mix well. Now add one or two drops of 1% bleaching powder solution (hypochlorite), from a dropper, and mix by decanting. The appearance of a blue colour in the chloroform layer (at the bottom of the tube) indicates the presence of indican. If no colour appears after waiting a few minutes, add more acid and repeat the decanting. If no colour results, add more acid and a drop of bleaching powder and mix again. The addition of excessive amounts of bleaching powder solution will dissolve out the colour. In some animals, a lot of acid may be required to produce a satisfactory result owing to the high buffering capacity of the urine.

In canine urine, the presence of indican indicates a degree of alimentary stasis or intestinal toxaemia, for example in constipation or intestinal obstruction.

URINE DEPOSITS

The microscopic examination of spun deposits is often omitted in practice, which is very unfortunate. My personal opinion is that all routine urine analyses should include a deposit examination or, at the least, those samples in which chemical changes have been detected, e.g. protein is present, should be examined.

The urine sample should be centrifuged for 5 minutes at 2000 rpm. The supernatant is removed and an aliquot of the deposit is then transferred to a microscope slide and a cover slip applied. The deposit is examined as an unstained preparation using x 10 or x 40 objectives.

Alternatively a staining procedure may be employed to facilitate the differentiation of various cellular elements in a deposit, for example Kova-stain (BCL) may be used.

Whichever method is used some experience and tuition is required in order to become proficient at the examination of urine deposits. A diagrammatic representation of the commoner cells and crystalline or amorphous deposits seen in urine, is shown in Figures 3.1 and 3.2. Bacteria will only be motile in fresh unpreserved samples.

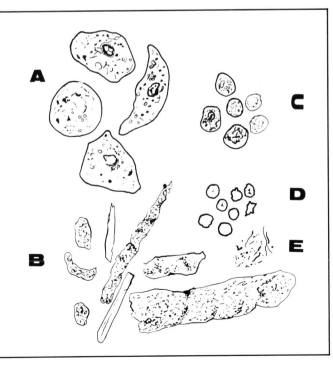

Figure 3.1
Cellular or protein derived
urine deposits
(approximately to scale)

A = Epithelial cells
B = various granular or hyaline casts;
    cellular casts are not illustrated
C = leucocytes
D = erythcocytes
E = bacteria.

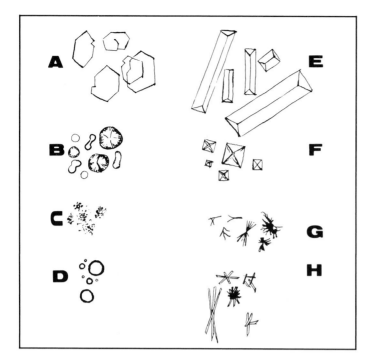

Figure 3.2
Crystalline or non cellular
urine deposits. (size approximate)

A = cystine
B = carbonates
C = amorphous urates or phosphates
D = fat globules
E = triple phosphates
    (ammonium magnesium phosphate)
F = oxalate
G = bilirubin (brown/orange colour)
H = bi urates or stellar phosphates.

The cells are of three types: —

a. epithelial cells from various parts of the urinary tract;

b. leucocytes which are smaller and have granular contents and

c. erythrocytes, which are the smallest of all, have no visible contents and may be crenated.

Casts containing obvious cellular material are only seen in very acute nephritis. The crystalline deposits illustrated are not to scale as crystal size varies enormously but generally speaking triple phosphate (Struvite) crystals are large; oxalate, cystine and carbonate crystals are easily seen, while amorphous urates or phosphates are so small that their individual structure cannot be determined.

Urinary calculi can be identified by their physical shape and size but confirmation of their chemical structure relies on stone analysis kits which are available commercially e.g. Merck Diagnostics.

INTERPRETATION OF RESULTS

It is most important to look at all the results of a urine analysis before coming to any conclusion and probably even more important to relate the urine analysis results to the history and clinical signs displayed by the patient and to any other test results. It is unwise to take individual urine analysis results too literally; for example, the fact that a dog urine contains bilirubin is of itself a valueless piece of information. If, however, bile salts are also present in quantity, the animal shows clinical signs relating to liver dysfunction and later is shown to have appropriate abnormal serum enzyme levels then the interpretation is totally different.

Despite these reservations I will, in this article, deal with the interpretation of each estimation separately in order to make matters as clear as possible.

CHEMICAL TESTS

Specific gravity

Normal range 1.015 — 1.045 (mean 1.020)

The specific gravity of a single sample is of little importance. A consistently low specific gravity indicates an inability of the kidney to concentrate urine, as in chronic interstitial nephritis or diabetes insipidus. A consistently high specific gravity indicates the presence of substances such as glucose, as in diabetes mellitus or may indicate disease conditions such as congestive cardiac failure.

pH

Normal range (carnivores) 5—7

Alkaline urine may be encountered in stale samples in animals with bacterial infections of the urinary tract e.g. cystitis and occasionally in animals on non meat diets. Excessively low pH may be seen in starvation.

Protein

Protein is normally absent from the urine but its presence is not necessarily a sign of disease (functional proteinuria). On the other hand, its presence may have marked clinical significance (organic proteinuria).

> **Functional proteinuria:** This term is applied to those cases in which the urinary protein appears to have no pathological significance. It is invariably intermittent. Thorough clinical examination of the patient and complete urine analysis reveal no evidence of renal disease or involvement of any part of the genito-urinary tract. It may be seen after severe exertion, severe exposure or excessive feeding.

> **Organic proteinuria:** This is usually persistent and more severe than the functional type. Clinical examination and complete urine analysis provide other evidence of renal disease. Proteinuria may be derived from inflammation of the bladder, urethra or prostate. Large amounts of protein are present in acute nephritis, glomerulo-nephritis and nephroses. Moderate to small amounts are present in chronic interstitial nephritis. Protein may occur in the urine in acute febrile conditions, in anaemia, in passive congestion due to cardiac disease and as a sequel to many acute diseases. Contamination of the urine sample with discharge from prepuce or vagina will give positive protein tests, e.g. oestrus, metritis, pyometra, balanitis.

Blood

Normally blood is absent from urine. When present, it may occur either as intact cells or as free haemoglobin, viz:

> **Haematuria:** The presence of red blood cells in the urine caused by inflammation or injury of any part of the tract leading to haemorrhage. Causes include actual trauma, calculi, chemical irritants, acute septicaemic conditions, neoplasms and parasites. The exact source of whole blood cannot be decided from examination of the urine alone.

> **Haemoglobinuria:** The presence of pigment with few, if any, red blood cells in the urine. Usually follows haemoglobinaemia, the principal causes of which are blood parasites, e.g. piroplasmosis or massive intravascular haemolysis caused by other factors. Red blood cells and free haemoglobin may be found together in cases of acute nephritis, pyelitis, cystitis and urethritis.

Bilirubin (bile pigments)

Normally, bile pigments (conjugated bilirubin) are absent from urine. Small quantities are sometimes detectable in normal dog urine, but in these cases bile **salts** are absent. The presence of bile pigments in demonstrable quantities is most commonly due to obstruction of the bile ducts, disease or dysfunction of the liver or following excessive haemolysis. Positive results may also follow chlorpromazine therapy. Unconjugated bilirubin does not pass the renal filter and will not be seen in urine.

Bile salts

Normally, bile salts (the sodium salts of glycocholic acid and taurocholic acid) are absent from urine. Their presence is indicative of similar conditions to those noted under bile pigments.

Urobilinogen

Urobilinogen is formed in the intestine by the bacterial reduction of conjugated bilirubin and is mostly excreted in the faeces. When large amounts of conjugated bilirubin pass into the intestine, some of the urobilinogen formed is re-absorbed and either processed by the liver or excreted in the urine. Thus, high urine urobilinogen levels may be seen in cases of haemolytic disease. In some cases of liver dysfunction, the liver may be unable to process urobilinogen from the portal circulation and it is excreted in the urine. Urobilinogen is only detected satisfactorily in **fresh** urine samples and its practical value in veterinary medicine is much less than in the human field.

Indican

Indole, a product of intestinal breakdown of albuminous substances, is absorbed into the blood and oxidised in the tissues to indoxyl, which combines with potassium sulphate and is eliminated in the urine as an ethereal sulphate (indican).

In canine urine, the presence of indican indicates a degree of alimentary stasis or intestinal toxaemia, for example, in constipation or intestinal obstruction.

Glucose

The renal threshold for glucose is 8—10 mmol/l. Normal urine has no reducing properties. In a very small proportion of animals, the renal threshold for glucose is abnormally low. In pregnant lactating animals, traces of sugar (lactose) may be found in the urine. Some drugs, if present in large amounts, may cause a slight reduction of Benedict's reagent, e.g. chloral hydrate and salicylates. Injury to the floor of the fourth ventricle causes glucosuria. Transitory glucosuria may arise from fear, excitement, anxiety — stimulation of the adrenal sympathetic mechanism. It may also occur after exercise, during pregnancy and after the alimentary or parenteral administration of glucose. In terminal toxaemia, glucose will appear in the urine. In diabetes mellitus, a considerable amount of glucose is present in the urine. The detection of glucose in the urine of a dog should be followed by an estimation of **blood** glucose and by repeated urine analysis to ensure it is not a transitory phenomenon.

Ketone bodies

Ketone bodies are normally absent from urine. Their presence is usually due to a derangement in fat metabolism and deficiency of usable carbohydrate. In dogs, ketone bodies are found in the urine in cases of diabetes mellitus. (Ketone bodies will also appear in the urine in cases of advanced diabetes mellitus.) Ketone bodies may also appear in the urine during starvation. The ketone bodies of significance are acetone, aceto-acetic (diacetic) acid and beta-hydroxybutyric acid. Urine is not the most reliable fluid to use for ketone body detection as the kidney concentrates ketones and false high results may occur. In cases of ketonuria, it is essential to undertake blood glucose assays.

Bacteria

Some bacteria (gram negative) can convert nitrate to nitrite in urine. The tests detect nitrite and, when positive, indicate the presence of a bacterial infection within the urinary tract. A negative result does not indicate that bacteria are absent because a) some bacteria are unable to reduce nitrates, and b) unless the urine is retained for four hours in the bladder, there is insufficient time for the reduction to occur. Equally, bacteria multiplying in a voided urine sample may be capable of reducing nitrate to nitrite thus simulating the result obtained in genuine infection.

This test should, therefore, be performed on fresh urine, preferably the first sample in the morning, collected into clean containers. It is used as a preliminary screening test when urinary infections are suspected.

MICROSCOPIC EXAMINATION OF DEPOSITS

(See Figures 3.1 and 3.2)

Leucocytes

Leucocytes may be detected using commercial tests or by direct microscopy. Leucocytes will occur in increased numbers (>1 cell per high power field or 10 cells per μl) in any inflammatory or infected condition anywhere within the urinary tract. They may or may not be accompanied by bacteria. Contamination with preputial or vaginal discharges may be a source of leucocytes unrelated to the urinary tract. Epithelial cells are shed in small amounts into normal urine but excessive numbers are indicative of an inflammatory reaction within the urinary tract. Large epithelial cells tend to come from the bladder and small ones from the kidney but this is by no means invariably so.

Bacteria

The significance of bacteria in a deposit depends on the technique employed in obtaining the sample and on the age of the sample. Contamination of samples is the commonest source of bacteria in urine. To avoid contamination, use sterile catheters and bottles. Bacteriological examination is warranted if the clinical findings and the other evidence suggest the presence of infection in the urinary tract, e.g. in addition to the bacteria there are large numbers of leucocytes in the deposit. For microbiological details see page 104.

Casts

These are formed by coagulation of albuminous material within the collecting tubules of the kidney. When present in large numbers and associated with proteinuria, they are an indication of overt renal disease. The number seen per microscope field will depend on how dilute the urine sample was and in many cases of chronic uncompensated renal disease, a few casts is a significant finding. Casts are classified according to their microscopical appearance as hyaline, granular, epithelial, blood, leucocyte or waxy. Granular forms are the commonest type.

Hyaline: Transparent refractile consisting entirely of protein. Found in many instances of renal disease, but may occur in small numbers in normal urine. All other casts are basically hyaline casts with different types of cells or other material present.

Waxy: More highly refractile than hyaline casts and have a dull, opaque lustre. They are most frequently associated with nephroses and are not common.

Granular: Contain either fine or coarse granules composed of various proteins. Seen in the later stages of acute and sub-acute nephritis and older-standing cases. These are the commonest form of casts encountered in dogs with renal disease.

Cellular: Have a hyaline or granular core to which the cells adhere. Most frequently associated with the more acute forms of renal disease. Cells may be epithelial or red or white blood cells.

Crystalline and amorphous deposits

These are common and usually of no pathological significance. The reaction of the urine influences the nature and type of such deposits. Only if calculi are present are the crystals of significance. In **alkaline** urine, phosphates and carbonates are often found.

Crystals are not commonly found in **acid** urine, but calcium oxalate, uric acid and urate crystals may sometimes occur. In dogs, cystine crystals appear in cystinuria which is an inherited condition. Calculi formation is common in this condition and hence the presence of cystine crystals in urine is of importance. The significance of other crystalline material has to be assessed in the light of all the other available information.

ADDITIONAL INFORMATION

The suppliers of reagents and equipment relating to urine analysis are listed on page 145.

CHAPTER 4

TRANSUDATIVE AND EXUDATIVE FLUIDS

D. L. Doxey B.V.M.& S., Ph.D., M.R.C.V.S.

INTRODUCTION

Fluids accumulate for a variety of reasons at sites where little fluid is normally present and the examination of these transudative or exudative fluids can be extremely valuable in certain circumstances. This procedure is, unfortunately, often neglected or not even considered by practitioners enquiring into why large volumes of fluid are accumulating in various parts of the body.

If fluid is known to to have gathered, for instance, in the abdominal cavity or in a joint, it does seem an eminently suitable idea to remove some of the fluid and examine it to ascertain what type of fluid it is and see whether it will guide you to the cause of the problem. In many cases I have encountered, this simple principle is ignored and when laboratory based tests are undertaken by the practitioner, they cover almost everything except the analysis of the abnormal fluid. I was recently involved with a dog exhibiting gross ascites which was suspected as being due to cardiac malfunction. Sodium, potassium and urea levels in serum and routine haematology had been requested to help with the diagnosis but no ascitic fluid was analysed. The animal turned out to have an abdominal tumour!

I cannot stress strongly enough that the laboratory assessment of abnormal fluids should head your list of priorities when there is any direct evidence to show that fluid has accumulated in an abnormal site.

The fluids which are likely to gather or show alterations are as follows:-

>Pleural and peritoneal fluids
>
>Synovial fluids
>
>Cerebro spinal fluids
>
>Other sites e.g. salivary cyst.

The fluid withdrawn from these sites may be of two types.

>**Transudates** — that is a fluid which has accumulated passively and **exudates**, which are actively produced as the result of an inflammatory reaction. In addition there are also fluids known as modified transudates which fall somewhere between the two types. It must be remembered that the composition of these fluids is not static but will change from hour to hour and a transudate may become an exudate, or vice versa.

SAMPLE COLLECTION

Aseptic precautions are essential, even when bacteriological examination is not contemplated, in order to ensure that tapping the affected area does not introduce infection. In all cases, the puncture site should be shaved and cleaned and local anaesthetic applied if required. Sterile needles (usually 18—22 gauge) and sterile syringes, should be employed. With abdominal paracentesis, the needle is inserted close to the midline, in front of the umbilicus. Ensure that no blood, due to skin puncture, enters the sample.

Thoracic fluid is removed from the intercostal space between ribs 7 and 8 in the lower third of the chest, keeping close to the anterior edge of the rib. The volume of fluid removed may vary from a few millilitres to several hundred, depending on the case. The site of penetration in a swollen joint will depend on the individual joint. The volume of fluid obtained can be anything up to about 5 mls.

For cerebrospinal fluid collection, general anaesthesia is usually required and one of two collection sites can be used; the cisterna magna at the atlanto-occipital articulation, or the spinal subarachnoid space in the lumbar region. In either site, the fluid should be removed slowly. The volume of fluid removed should not exceed 5 ml in a big dog and in cats, it is dangerous to remove more than 1 ml.

Once fluid has been removed from whatever site, it can be treated in several ways. A proportion, or in the case of small samples where bacteriology is not required, all the sample, should be placed in EDTA using the same anticoagulant ratio as for blood (see page 56). With small sample volumes, it will be necessary to use paediatric containers. Any fluid for bacteriological assessment, should be placed in a sterile heparinised container. EDTA is not suitable for bacterial or viral isolation, but is preferred for cellular identification.

If samples are placed in containers without anticoagulant, there is a chance of them coagulating if their protein content is very high. Clotted samples are not suitable for laboratory analysis.

LABORATORY METHODS

The tests undertaken are uniform irrespective of where the sample was obtained except for synovial fluid on which mucin clot tests may be performed.

Visual appraisal is important. In general, clear yellow or water-like fluids are likely to be transudates and cloudy or discoloured fluids, exudative in nature. Visual appraisal must be followed by further tests — on its own it is not reliable.

Specific gravity. The same methods itemised under urine analysis can be used. A refractometer is the best method.

Protein. This test is one which helps to distinguish transudative and exudative fluids and should be undertaken when possible. A specially calibrated refractometer can be used or a technique such as Biuret, which requires a colorimetric reading, can be employed. It would not be considered normal practice to undertake electrophoresis on these fluids, but it can be done in exceptional circumstances.

Lipids. Total lipids can be undertaken using kit techniques such as the one produced by BCL.

Cell counts. The manual haematological techniques described on page 57 are used for total and differential cell counts. It is possible to use electronic counters to do total red and white cell counts, but the results are not always reliable on exudative fluid because of the cell clumping and distortion which occurs. It is best to use a manual technique for exudative fluids but in the case of white cell counts, substitute physiological saline for the 2% acetic acid normally used in white cell diluting fluid. This is to avoid problems with protein coagulation.

Differentials may be prepared as described on page 61 after centrifugation and the deposit is used to prepare the smear. Alternatively, a cytospin technique may be used if the necessary equipment is available. (Shandon Ltd.).

Differential counts are not always easy because there is often very marked cell distortion, clumping and disruption as a result of inflammatory reactions. In a few cases, it is impossible to identify all the cells and generalisations have to be made. It is of vital importance to record all abnormal cells especially when neoplasia is suspected.

Microbiology.

The techniques applicable are described on page 106.

Special tests.

In the case of **synovial fluid** the mucin clot test can be employed.

Spin the sample and place 0.2 ml supernatant in a tube. Add to this 0.8 ml distilled water and 1 drop of acetic acid diluted 1:25 with water before use. Stir well and examine for clot formation. Evaluate the clot formed as good, fair or poor. Fair or poor clots indicate synovial abnormalities.

In the case of **cerebrospinal fluid** a test for **globulin** can be undertaken, (Pandy's test). Pandy's fluid is 7% phenol.

Add 1 drop CSF to 0.5 ml Pandy's fluid and look for turbidity. The greater the turbidity, the higher the globulin level.

INTERPRETATION OF RESULTS

The generally recognised definition of transudates and exudates is given below.

Transudates

These are fluids which accumulate in abnormal amounts as a result of the passive leakage of fluids from the circulation into the cavity. They have the following characteristics:

1. Clear, transparent, odourless fluid.
2. A specific gravity of less than 1.018.
3. Protein content of 5—30 g/litre (mainly albumin unless the liver is diseased, when globulins predominate).
4. Total lipids less than 1.5 g/litre.
5. Electrolytes, glucose, urea and other non-protein nitrogen compounds present in the same quantities as in plasma.
6. Cells are infrequently present and are almost exclusively mononuclear.
   (Total usually less than 1×10^9/litre and neutrophils less than 5%).

Exudates

These are abnormal and are actively produced by a reaction such as inflammation. They have the following characteristics:

1. Clear-opaque fluids varying greatly in colour and often having an offensive odour.
2. Specific gravity is above 1.018 and may exceed 1.026. They may be watery or thick and turgid.
3. Protein content exceeds 30 g/litre. Fibrinogen or fibrin may be present when capillary damage is severe and these fluids may clot very quickly.
4. Lipids are often high (above 3.3 g/litre in pleural exudates) and said to be high in cases of malignancy.
5. Electrolytes, urea and other non-protein nitrogen compounds are present in the same quantities as plasma, but glucose may be low if glucose utilising bacteria are present.
6. Cells are present in quantity and many will be neutrophils. Counts as high as 100×10^9/l may be seen.
7. Bacteria are often present and fungi may be seen.

The figures given here are not sacrosanct and variations will occur; for example, the protein content may exceed 30 g/l but the white cell count may not be elevated. Fluids of this type are generally referred to as modified transudates.

Transudates accumulate passively in conditions such as cardiac failure, cirrhosis of the liver or when serum albumin levels are extremely low. In such cases, pleural or peritoneal accumulations will be likely and dependent oedema may also be present.

Exudates are positively produced by an inflammatory infective or neoplastic process which actively drives protein into the affected area and brings forth a cellular response to the causal agent or agents.

In joint lesions, the accumulation of fluid without obvious cellular response, may follow closed traumatic damage. In the cerebro spinal fluid, obvious cellular responses are relatively uncommon and confined mainly to conditions such as overt meningitis.

It is important to remember that these abnormal fluid accumulations are in a constant dynamic state of flux and their composition will change hourly. A transudate may become an exudate or an exudate will change its character and composition as the clinical disease progresses or regresses. It is always useful to take serial samples to assess these changes in fluid composition which will enable the clinician to reach a more precise diagnosis and prognosis.

It is essential to relate the laboratory results to the duration and type of illness being shown by the patient. The number and type of cells in the fluid is also of great importance and, whenever possible, identification should be made. Remember that inflammatory cells may resemble immature neoplastic cells and care should be taken to distinguish them whenever possible. However, if you see large numbers of large, basophilic cells, especially if they occur in groups or clumps and have vacuolations or prominent nucleoli, neoplasia should be suspected. Absolute confirmation may require laparotomy and biopsy.

In the case of leucocytes, the type of cell present is recorded. Neutrophils in their various forms indicate inflammation. Histiocytes and macrophages are likely to be present in chronic inflammatory lesions, while excessive lymphocytes are often related to lymphoid neoplasia. Eosinophils and basophils may be associated with allergic reactions but, in my experience, the presence of large numbers of these cells, especially in cats, may be associated with neoplasia. Tumour cells are often impossible to identify specifically and the site of the original lesion will have to be sought by other diagnostic methods, e.g. X-rays.

If the erythrocytes appear in the fluid, ensure these are not there as a result of blood vessel puncture during sampling before ascribing them to pathological haemorrhage.

In a few instances, specific diagnostic information may be revealed by fluid examination; for example, chyle may appear due to thoracic duct rupture. In such a case, the fluid has a 'milky' appearance and the presence of fat can be demonstrated by dropping fluid onto a piece of absorbent paper which will become translucent.

In feline infectious peritonitis, the character of the fluid is often typical with low cell counts, lack of bacteria but high specific gravity (1.025—1.045) in conjunction with protein levels of 80 g/l or more. Electrophoresis of fluid and the patient's plasma will give almost identical results in such cases.

In the case of fluid accumulations which are thought to be due to specific causes, other laboratory tests may be appropriate. If, for example, bladder rupture is suspected, the estimation of urea on aspirated abdominal fluid should be compared with the animal's blood urea level. The fluid urea level will be grossly in excess of blood level if the bladder has ruptured.

OTHER INFORMATION

Apparatus and consumables suitable for use in the examination of fluids are itemised on page 145.

A list of appropriate suppliers is given on page 146

FURTHER READING

CAMPBELL, T. W. (1988). *Avian haematology and cytology.* Iowa State University Press.
COX, H. S. (1968). *Medical Cyto Technology.* Butterworths, London.

CHAPTER 5

HAEMATOLOGY

D. L. Doxey B.V.M. & S., Ph.D., M.R.C.V.S.

INTRODUCTION

Haematology has two main purposes in veterinary practice:

1. Confirming the diagnosis of specific blood disorders.
2. Assistance in the diagnosis of disease conditions which, although not of haematological origin, do cause appreciable non-specific changes in the distribution of blood cells.

SPECIFIC BLOOD DISORDERS

Irrespective of whether the pathological process affects the red or the white cells, the practitioner will be looking for known changes which have been clearly shown to be associated with specific conditions, e.g. neoplastic lymphocytes in lymphosarcoma, *Haemobartonella felis* in feline infectious anaemia or lack of platelets in thrombocytopenia. If these known changes can be demonstrated, a tentative diagnosis can be confirmed by haematology, in fact, in some cases it is the only way of confirming your clinical suspicions.

NON-SPECIFIC BLOOD CHANGES

Most clinical cases in which haematology has a diagnostic role fall into this category. The disease conditions are numerous. Haematological changes may vary from clearly significant cellular variations to barely perceptible changes which yield no clear conclusion. In this non-specific context, haematology is used as a general guide to detect changes in the ratio and number of blood cells. The results can then be applied in general terms to the clinical case, e.g. if total white cell count is raised due to neutrophilia, the presence of inflammation is revealed by the tests but not the precise cause or site of inflammation.

Haematolgical tests are often used in conjunction with other types of investigation, i.e. biochemical or bacteriological tests, and their diagnostic importance will vary with the type of case under examination.

The success or failure of haematology as an aid to diagnosis will depend on the clinician's ability to employ the techniques correctly. Successful use of haematology depends largely on the clinician's ability to select suitable clinical material. Significant results should not be expected in more than 50% of cases if haematology is used on a guesswork basis, i.e. employed because you cannot think of anything else to do. Correct selection depends on meeting the following criteria.

1. A complete clinical examination preceding the use of tests.
2. The clinician should have some idea of the type of pathological process involved.
3. The test(s) selected must have relevance to the clinical signs.
4. The suspected condition must be known to produce some haematological changes in the majority of instances.
5. The duration and severity of the condition must be taken into account.
6. The species of animal involved must be considered.

The selection of haematological tests which will be useful in the diagnosis of disease, is not easy. It requires a reasonable degree of knowledge of the subject, and is not infallible. If you remember that haematology is not useful in all diseases and employ it only in carefully screened and selected cases, then the results can be encouraging and helpful. If you use tests at random, without any selection procedures, the results will be poor, unhelpful or even misleading. Haematology is basically a screening technique.

SAMPLE COLLECTION

Table 5.1

Species	Site	Needle Gauge
Dog	Cephalic, saphenous or jugular vein	20−22
Cat	Cephalic, saphenous or jugular vein	22−24
Rabbit	Ear vein	22−24
Guinea pig	Ear vein, cardiac puncture*	20−22
Mouse	Tail vein, cardiac puncture*	23−25
Hamster	Cardiac puncture*	22−24

*Cardiac puncture is done under light anaesthesia.

Samples must be collected correctly if test results are to be valid.

In all cases, irrespective of the tests envisaged, the sample should be taken using dry, sterile apparatus, i.e. syringe and needle. The needle puncture site should be clipped and swabbed prior to sampling. Various sites can be used depending on the species of animal (Table 5.1).

Use minimum suction when withdrawing samples. Excess suction, wet equipment or squirting blood violently through fine-bore needles can all cause haemolysis of samples. Vacutainers or similar equipment also tend to cause haemolysis in some animals due to the effects of excessive suction, although this can be overcome to some extent by using the paediatric version.

After collection, blood must be prevented from clotting. This can be achieved in various ways, depending on the estimations required.

i)   Dipotassium sequestrene (EDTA) anticoagulant (2.5 mg/5 ml blood) is the method of choice for all routine haematological estimations. Ready prepared plastic bottles or vacutainers containing EDTA can be purchased and should be filled to the level indicated on the bottle or tube.

ii) Potassium oxalate (2-3 mg/ml blood) should be used if coagulation tests are required. This anticoagulant is not suitable for routine haematology. 3.8% sodium citrate can also be used for the same purposes as oxalate and is preferred in most instances. Heparin is not a good anticoagulant for haematology as it induces cellular distortion after only short periods of contact.

In all cases where anticoagulant is used, thoroughly mix the blood and anticoagulant to prevent clotting. Whenever possible , make certain that the blood : anticoagulant ratio is correct, i.e. do not put small amounts of blood into large amounts of anticoagulant, otherwise cell distortion occurs and red cell indices, in particular, may be altered. Contact with anticoagulant, even EDTA, will, after three days at room temperature, induce progressive and often marked cellular distortions and even haemolysis. It is consequently of importance to either examine samples as soon after collection as possible or to keep samples at 4° C until they can be processed.

LABORATORY METHODS

RED CELL INDICES

Under this heading can be grouped several estimations, all of which measure different aspects of the red cell population. Most commonly employed estimations are total red cell count, packed cell volume, haemoglobin content and reticulocyte count. From these results, the corpuscular values can be calculated. For practical purposes, the packed cell volume and haemoglobin estimations are the most reproducible and accurate techniques for anyone who only undertakes haematology occasionally. Cellular counts, especially total red (or white) cell counts, are prone to considerable errors in unskilled hands and are only recommended for use in practice laboratories employing trained technicians or experienced staff.

Total red cell count

Two methods are available. Manual techniques are used in small laboratories where estimations are undertaken infrequently and electronic cell counter techniques used in larger laboratories where red cell counts are carried out every day. It has become increasingly feasible in the past decade for large practices to afford and fully utilise electronic cell counters and now instruments employing buffy coat analysis are available for smaller laboratories.

i) Manual technique

Since the advent of AIDS mouth pipetting in laboratories is considered undesirable and the traditional red and white cell pipettes employing suction tubes are no longer used. Automatic pipettes for small volumes or pre-set dispensers for larger volumes are now standard practice. The diluting fluid consists of 3% sodium citrate (99ml) plus 40% formalin (1ml).

Method: Use an automatic pipette and an improved Neubauer haemocytometer. Place the coverslip firmly onto the haemocytometer. Mix the blood gently and carefully place 20 ml of diluting fluid into a container (an automatic dispenser can be used for this job). Take up 0.1 ml (100µl) of blood and wipe the automatic pipette tip clean.

Add the blood to the diluting fluid. Ensure that all the blood is dispersed by drawing fluid in and out until the pipette tip is clean. This gives a dilution of 1 : 200.

Put a lid on the container and mix the sample thoroughly.

Take an aliquot using a capillary tube. Place the tip of the capillary tube against the edge of the counting chamber coverslip and fill the counting area in a controlled way. Allow the cells to settle for 3 minutes and then count five of the squares in the central area (Figure 5.1, R) under either x 10 or x 40 objectives.

Calculation: Number of cells in five squares (80 small squares) divided by 100 = cells x 10 ^{12}/l.

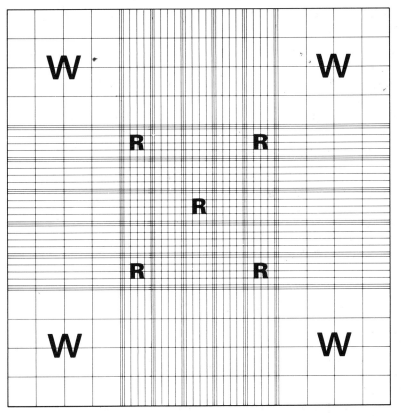

Figure 5.1

Technique accuracy: The technique requires practice and should be undertaken carefully and quietly. It is not the sort of technique one can stop in the middle to answer the telephone! A skilled technician undertaking the estimation regularly should have an error of less than $\pm$ 5%. In unskilled hands, especially if the test is hurried, the error can exceed $\pm$ 50%.

Time taken to undertake one estimation — approximately 8 minutes.

ii) Electronic cell counter

A variety of models are on the market and apparatus suitable for general practice are available from amongst others, Becton Dickinson, Clandon and Coulter. The following remarks apply to the Clandon Cell Dyn 800.

Special diluents (Haemocell isotonic diluent) are used. Place 40 μl (0.04 ml) of blood in 10 ml of diluent and mix. Transfer 40 μl of mixture into a further 10 ml of Haemocell to give a final dilution of 1 : 62500. Use this for counting using calibration or discriminator settings on the machine appropriate to the species involved (e.g. dog = 30, cat = 15). Always perform counts in duplicate.

Technique accuracy: The error should be $\pm$ 2%. The error with this technique is not the same as the error for a manual count as the diluent as well as the principles involved are different — manual technique counts cells, electronic technique counts particles. Consequently, the results obtained from the same sample will depend on the technique used; usually the higher counts are obtained with the electronic method, although the differences are not clinically significant. Time taken to undertake one estimation is approximately 8 minutes. This is markedly reduced per sample when several samples are assayed concurrently.

Packed cell volume

Three methods — centrifugation (Wintrobe method), microhaematocrits of various types, the electronic counter and buffy coat analysis.

i) Centrifugation (Wintrobe method)

Method: 1 ml of blood is required. A Wintrobe haematocrit tube is filled to the 100 mark with well mixed blood, using a Pasteur pipette. The pipette is pushed to the bottom of the Wintrobe tube and then slowly withdrawn as the blood is introduced into the tube. Care must be taken to avoid air bubbles. Spin the tube at 3,000 rpm for one hour in an ordinary balanced centrifuge. Read the result from the graduations on the tube.

Technique accuracy: Error less than $\pm$ 2%. Time taken — one hour.

ii) Microhaematocrit centrifugation

Method: 3—4 drops of blood are required. This technique employs a special centrifuge (Hawksley & Sons Ltd). Other mini centrifuges are now available to undertake these procedures.

Mix the sample thoroughly.

Take a special capillary tube and dip one end into the blood, allowing the tube to fill by capillary attraction to three-quarters of its length.

Wipe the outside of the tube clean.

Seal the unfilled end in a bunsen flame, taking care not to scorch the blood. (The end can be sealed with special filler (Hawksley). Other sealants or plastic tube caps can also be purchased (Critocaps, BCL.)).

Place the tube in the centrifuge, sealed end outwards. Spin for 5 minutes.

Technique accuracy: Method is rapid; accurate to $\pm$ 1% and requires less blood than the Wintrobe method. Main disadvantage is the special apparatus required.

iii) Electronic counter

Very accurate but costs may be prohibitive unless laboratory throughput is considerable. Attachments can be purchased for several counters to allow PCV values to be calculated automatically and now buffy coat analysis can also be used (see total white cell count).

Haemoglobin estimation

Several methods — cyanmethaemoglobin, alkaline haematin and electronic counter.

i) Cyanmethaemoglobin

The principle relies on conversion of haemoglobin to methaemoglobin to cyanmethaemoglobin followed by colorimetric measurement.

Method:

Modified Drabkin's reagent (pH 7.0 — 7.4)

Potassium ferricyanide	200 mg
Potassium cyanide	50 mg
Potassium dihydogen phosphate	140 mg
* Nonidet P40 (Shell Chemical Company)	1 ml
Water	to 1 litre

* Detergents speed up the reaction time. Ready prepared solutions can be purchased (BDH).

Add 0.02 ml blood to 5 ml modified Drabkin's reagent.

Stopper and invert several times.

Stand for 3 minutes and read in a colorimeter using a yellow-green filter (Ilford 624) or at 540 nanometres in a spectrophotometer and compare with a known haemoglobin or commercial cyanmethaemoglobin standard against a reagent blank.

Time taken for one estimation is 15 minutes.

Technique accuracy: The error is $\pm$ 5%.

ii) Alkaline haematin

Haemoglobin is converted to alkaline haematin and measured colorimetrically.

Method: Add 0.05 ml blood to 4.95 ml 10 mmol/l sodium hydroxide in a test tube, heat for 5 minutes in a boiling water bath and then cool rapidly in cold water.

When cold, and within half an hour of boiling, read on a colorimeter using a yellow-green filter (Ilford 624) or at 540 nanometers. Gibson & Harrison's artificial standard is boiled and cooled alongside the unknown. This standard equals 16 g of haemoglobin per dl of blood. By comparing the colorimeter readings of the standard and the unknown, the haemoglobin content of the unknown can be determined, e.g.

$$\frac{\text{Reading of unknown}}{\text{Reading of standard}} \times 16 = \text{haemoglobin in g/dl blood}$$

If foetal haemoglobin is present, boil for 15 minutes to ensure that all foetal haemoglobin is converted.

Time for one estimation is 12 minutes.

Technique accuracy: The error is $\pm$ 5%.

iii) Electronic counter

Attachments to allow haemoglobin to be calculated automatically can be obtained for several electronic counters.

The error is about $\pm$ 2%.

Reticulocyte counts

Reticulocytes are stained supra vitally, that is, live cells are incubated with a dye. They are not stained by the methods used for blood smears.

Reticulocytes, when stained with brilliant cresyl blue, have a distinct reticular pattern. Such cells appear in large numbers during the recovery phase following anaemia and their presence can be used as a guide to the ability of the bone marrow to produce new cells. Reticulocytes are seen in the dog, cat (normal values less than 1%). In other species listed in Table 5.2, normal values are 2—4% and in the hamster up to 10%.

Method: Stain composed of

3% sodium citrate	20 ml
0.85% sodium chloride	80 ml
brilliant cresyl blue	0.4 g
filtered just prior to use.	

2 ml of stain are placed in a centrifuge tube, 4-5 drops of blood are added, mixed and the tube is placed vertically in an incubator at 37° C for 30 minutes (one hour at room temperature).

Spin gently, decant the supernatant stain and resuspend the cells at the bottom of the tube.

Prepare the smears in the usual manner.

After the film has dried, count at least 1,000 cells under oil immersion objective and ascertain the number of reticulocytes present. Alternatively, find the mean number of cells in at least 10 microscope fields and then find out how many further fields have to be observed to detect 100 reticulocytes. From these findings, reticulocyte percentage can be deduced, i.e.

$$\frac{\text{Number of reticulocytes seen}}{\text{Total number of cells scanned}} \times 100 = \text{percentage}$$

One estimation would take 40 minutes (longer if at room temperature).

Technique accuracy: The greater the reticulocyte percentage the more accurate the technique. The greater number of cells counted, the more accurate the result. The method should give errors of $\pm$ 10% when reticulocyte percentage is above 5%. If reticulocyte percentage is between 1% and 5%, the error is $\pm$ 20%.

Corpuscular values

These are calculated from results of the total red cell count, packed cell volume and haemoglobin. Accuracy, and hence diagnostic usefulness, depends entirely on the accuracy of techniques from which they are calculated. Only if basic techniques are accurate can any reliance be placed on corpuscular values. The three corpuscular values referred to are as follows and are quoted in SI Units.

Mean cell volume (MCV) =

$$\frac{\text{Packed cell volume l/l} \times 1,000}{\text{Red cells} \times 10^{12}/l} = fl$$

Mean corpuscular haemoglobin (MCH) =

$$\frac{\text{Haemoglobin in g/dl} \times 10}{\text{Red cells} \times 10^{12}/l} = pg$$

Mean corpuscular haemoglobin concentration (MCHC) =

$$\frac{\text{Haemoglobin in g/dl}}{\text{Packed cell volume l/l}} = \text{g/dl}$$

Normal adult corpuscular values are as follows:

	MCV	MCH	MCHC
Dog	60–77	19–23	31–35
Cat	39–55	12.5–15.5	29–34

Sedimentation rate

Method: Fill a Wintrobe tube with blood, using a Pasteur pipette and taking care to avoid air bubbles.

Stand the tube vertically, in a special stand, for one hour at room temperature and then measure the distance the red cells have sedimented. The result should be corrected for packed cell volume because sedimentation increases as the packed cell volume decreases. Charts for this conversion have been published (Schalm 1986).

Sedimentation rate increases with increasing age of the sample.

Technique accuracy: Provided the blood : anticoagulant ratio is correct, and the sample has been thoroughly mixed, results are accurate.

WHITE CELL INDICES

The two estimations are total and differential white cell counts. It is important that these estimations are done together, as one without the other may give misleading results.

Total white cell count

Three methods are available — one manual, the electronic cell counter techniques and buffy coat analysis. The remarks made previously concerning the red cell count also apply to the total white cell count.

i) Manual technique. The diluting fluid consists of a 2% solution of acetic acid (99 ml to which is added 1 ml gentian violet).

Use an automatic pipette and improved Neubauer haemocytometer.

Place 2 ml diluting fluid into a container.

Take up 0.1 ml (100 μl) of blood in the pipette. Wipe the pipette tip and dispense blood into the diluting fluid. Place lid on the container and mix.

Final dilution 1 : 20.

The procedure after this is as described for the red cell count.

Count the cells in four large squares (Figure 5.1, W. page 57).

Total cells counted in four large squares, divided by 20 = cells 10^9/l.

Technique accuracy: See red cell count.

ii) Electronic cell counter. The remarks refer to the Clandon Cell-Dyn 800.

The first dilution described for the red cell count (page 58) is completed, e.g. $40\mu l$ in 10 ml Haemocell.

Mix and remove 40 μl for the red cell count.

Add 6 drops of a lysing agent (e.g. Haemolysin) and mix.

The red cells are lysed.

The final dilution is 1 : 250.

Place the container on the counter and undertake triplicate counts with the discriminator settings at 7 for all species.

Technique accuracy: See under total red cell count.

iii) Buffy coat analysis. Recently, an instrument designed for practice use on canine and feline samples and employing buffy coat analysis, has been introduced. (Becton Dickinson). This method involves taking up a mixed blood sample into a special large microhaematocrit tube containing a plastic float. The tube is then capped and placed in the centrifuge. After centrifugation for 5 minutes the various layers have separated within the tube. The tube is placed into the reading instrument and viewed through an eyepiece. The various layers are moved into view and 'read' by the instrument on the press of a button. When the scan is complete the machine will give a digital display of the results.

The following can be measured using this procedure. Packed cell volume, platelets, total white cell count, total and percentage granulocyte count and total and percentage mononuclear cell count.

The instrument is useful as a screening procedure in general practice but for PCV and total white cell counts is likely to have errors up to $\pm$ 10%. This is less accurate than advanced cell counters but then the price is considerably lower.

Differential white cell count.

The best smears are prepared using fresh blood but good results can be obtained from EDTA samples provided they are not too old. Preparation and staining of the smear are crucial and, if undertaken badly, the count results may be difficult to interpret. The following types are usualy defined in the dog and cat.

Neutrophils, mature	— nucleus U-shaped, thin or segmented
Neutrophils, immature	— nucleus U-shaped, thick not segmented.
Lymphocytes	
Monocytes	
Eosinophils	
Basophils	

In rabbits and guinea pigs, the neutrophil granules have eosinophilic staining properties and are called pseudo-eosinophils. In the hamster, the unsegmented neutrophil nucleus may be round like a doughnut.

Method: Use clean, grease-free slides.

Place a small drop of blood at one end of a glass slide.

Take a spreader slide (a glass slide with one end narrower than the other) and place the narrow end against the surface of the first slide at an angle of 40° in front of the drop of blood (Figure 5.2).

Draw the spreader slide back until the blood spreads out along the narrow edge.

Push the spreader slide steadily forward. This draws the blood along and spreads it out into a thin film.

Wave the smear in the air to dry it rapidly.

Smears made by this method should be thin and leave at least 1 mm between the edges of the smear and the slide. Never allow the smear to run over the edge of the slide.

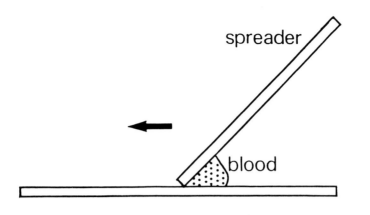

Figure 5.2

Several methods of staining are available, but the most commonly used is Leishman's stain. Smears are best stained shortly after preparation. If there is to be a delay, fix the smear in absolute methyl alcohol for one minute. This preserves the cells and staining can then be delayed without any risk of cellular degeneration.

Leishman's staining technique. Place smear (blood uppermost) on a staining rack over the sink.
Place enough concentrated stain on slide to cover it.
Leave for 2 minutes
Add twice the stain's volume of buffered distilled water (pH 6.8) and mix well.
Leave for 15 minutes.
Wash thoroughly with water and then allow smear to dry at room temperature.
Prepared glass slides on which dye has been coated are commercially available (Testsimplets BCL).
A drop of blood is placed on the prepared area, a coverslip applied and after 15 minutes the preparation is ready for examination under the microscope. This saves smearing and staining in the conventional manner for anyone who does not undertake the procedure regularly. They can also be used to stain other types of material, such as CSF or peritoneal fluid.

Technique accuracy: The greatest difficulty is accurate identification of various cell types. This is a procedure which requires initial tuition and considerable practice, but is made easier when the smears are well prepared and stained. Accuracy depends on familiarity and practice.

Buffy coat analysis can also be used for partial differential counts (see total WBC counts).

Demonstration of blood parasites

Haemobartonella felis causes anaemia in cats and is troublesome in some areas of the country. *Dirofilaria immitis* (heartworm) occurs in dogs in quarantine or in dogs which have been imported and whose quarantine period is completed. It is, consequently, unusual in Britain.

i) Haemobartonella felis. Blood films are prepared in the manner described previously. Staining is carried out using Giemsa stain.

Method: Fix smear with absolute methanol (2 minutes). Dilute Giemsa stain with buffered distilled water (pH 6.8) to a dilution of 1 : 10. Stain smear for 15 minutes.

Wash in water until film appears pink.

Dry and examine under oil immersion lens. Parasites appear as small, pleomorphic, round or rod-shaped bodies, staining purple and attached to the outside of the red cells. They can easily be confused with stain deposit and are not always detectable even in known positive cases.

H. felis can also be demonstrated using an acridine orange technique and fluorescent microscopy. This method is generally better at detecting low levels of infection than the Giesma technique.

Method: (Jahanmehr *et al,* 1987). The dye consists of 0.5 g Acridine Orange and 8.5 g of sodium chloride made up in 1 litre of distilled water.

Place 50 μl of fresh blood into a small clean test tube and add an equal volume of dye.

Mix for 2 minutes and then prepare blood smears in the normal way. Dry the smear as rapidly as possible and examine under oil immersion using incident ultra violet light.

With low levels of parasitaemia the dilution effect of adding dye can be eliminated by using prepared tubes in which the dye (25 μl at 1g/Litre concentration) has been dried by prior incubation at 37°C and to which the blood is then added and mixed.

Parasites fluoresce a green/yellow colour.

Technique accuracy: Difficult to assess as parasite numbers may be low and easily missed. Slides should be examined thoroughly before a negative finding is announced. A negative result is inconclusive.

ii) Dirofilaria immitis. Several methods available. A drop of blood can be placed on a slide and examined under a coverslip for signs of larval activity. Serum samples can also be used.

It is important to distinguish between *D. immitis* larvae, which have straight tails, and *Dipetalonema* spp, which are non-pathogenic and have curved tails. Several methods are available for this purpose (including commercially available kits made in America) but only two will be described here.

Method 1: Serum from about 3 ml of blood is placed in 5 cc of 2 — 5% acetic acid and centrifuged at 1,500 r.p.m. for 5 minutes. The supernatant is discarded and the sediment examined for the dead larvae.

Method 2: This involves forcing blood, collected in EDTA, through a 1μm pore size nucleopore filter, by means of a syringe. the filter can be examined unstained for the presence of microfilaria or it can be stained for acid phosphatase to help distinguish *D. immitis* from *Dipetalonema* spp. (Acevedo *et al,* 1981).

Technique accuracy: If larvae are present and all deposit is examined, the results should be satisfactory. A negative finding does not preclude the presence of microfilaria. See page 84 for further information.

Platelet count

Not a routine technique but very valuable especially in bleeding disorders.

Method: Diluting fluid is Baar's (J. Clin Path. 1 : 175 (1948).

Saponin (BDH)	...	0.25 g
Sodium citrate	...	3.50 g
40% formaldehyde	...	1.0 ml
Distilled water	...	100.0 ml

A half-thickness improved Neubauer haemocytometer is used which allows sufficient light to penetrate, but a full thickness haemocytometer can be employed. The technique is the same as for total white cell count (manual), i.e. 1 : 20 dilution.

Allow cells to settle for 30 minutes (inside a damp Petri dish to prevent evaporation) and then count five squares (Figure 5.1, R, page 57).

The number of platelets counted = cells x $10^9/1$.

Normal values in domestic animals range from 200 — 600 x $10^9/1$.

Technique accuracy: As for total red cell count.

Estimated time is 40 minutes (30 minutes is 'waiting time'). In large laboratories platelet counts are now undertaken using special electronic cell counters.

Clotting defects

The sophisticated human techniques, i.e. thromboplastin generation test, or factor VIII assay, are not feasible and often not appropriate in veterinary practice. Measurement of prothrombin time is a feasible and relatively simple laboratory test which can be undertaken with limited resources.

The measurement of the activated partial thromboplastin test is now feasible in practice as a kit technique is available.

Prothrombin time. This test is done using oxalated or citrated plasma. Never use plasma extracted from an EDTA sample. The test measures not only deficiencies of prothrombin but also factor V, VII and X deficiencies.

> **Method:** Place normal control plasma , patient's plasma and a source of brain thromboplastin* in a water bath and allow them to reach 37° C. Each estimation is done in triplicate.
>
> Place 0.1 ml of control plasma in each of three tubes. Allow the temperature to reach 37° C and then add 0.2 ml thromboplastin to the first tube. Start the stopwatch immediately.
>
> Either shake the tube gently in the water bath or move a wire loop up and down in the tube until a white clot of fibrin appears. Note the time taken.
>
> Repeat the procedure on the other tubes and test the patient's plasma in the same way. It is often easier to see the clot formation if the test is carried out in a small glass container holding water at 37° C in which the tube under test is suspended.
> Normal range for prothrombin time: 8—15 seconds.

$$\text{Prothrombin index} - \frac{\text{Normal prothrombin time} \times 100}{\text{Patient's prothrombin time}}$$

In cases of prothrombin deficiency, the prothrombin time will be increased. In total prothrombin deficiency, the plasma will never clot. Remember that clotting is also inhibited by Factor V, VII and X deficiency and that the presence of heparin will invalidate the results.

Technique accuracy: Accurate to within 1—2 seconds of the mean value and can be done in any practice.

* Brain thromboplastin with added calcium is available commercially. i.e. Simplastin (General Diagnostics), Calcium thromboplastin (BCL).

Activated partial thromboplastin test (APTT). This is a screening test used to detect the absence of coagulation factors in the intrinsic coagulation cascade e.g. factor VIII. The test will not detect platelet factor 3 nor will it tell you which factor is missing, only that one is absent.

> **Technique.** Reagents: 0.025 M calcium chloride.
> Platelin plus activator (General Diagnostics). This contains rabbit brain phospholipid as a source of factor 3 and a particulate activator, called celite, in a buffer.

Method.

1. Prewarm calcium chloride to 37° C in a water bath.

2. Label tubes patient and control.

3. Add 0.1 ml (100μl) patient plasma or control plasma to appropriate tube.
   Add 0.1 ml (100μl) platelin plus activator.

4. Incubate at 37° C for five minutes.

5. Add 0.1 ml (100 µl) 0.025 M calcium chloride and start a stop watch. Move a wire loop gently in the liquid.
6. Wait until a white clot forms on the loop. Stop the watch and record the time.

Normal control value: 14—25 seconds. Technique accuracy as for prothrombin time.

N.B. This test is sensitive to heparin and cannot, therefore, be undertaken on a heparinised sample. Other coagulation tests of value in practice are clotting time and clot retraction.

Whole blood clotting time. This is performed in small, (70mm x 9mm), scrupulously clean capped glass tubes (Lee and White method). 1 ml of fresh blood is introduced into the tube and the time taken from sample aspiration to clotting is recorded. It is essential that the test is undertaken at 37° C. A water bath is therefore required but, in emergencies, putting the tube in an inside pocket will suffice although the error thus introduced may exceed 20%. The normal value for dogs is less than 10 minutes.

Clot retraction. Place 5 ml of fresh blood in a glass test tube (preferably siliconised) containing a spiral wire and allow it to clot at 37° C. Incubate for a further hour and then remove the clot by means of the wire. Measure volume of fluid expressed from the clot i.e. 1 ml fluid removed from 5 ml blood represents a clot retraction of only 20%.

Alternatively, clotted blood can be left at room temperature and observed after several hours to see if the clot has retracted from the glass but, this is less satisfactory. Clot retraction is largely related to efficient platelet function.

Technique accuracy. Accuracy is related to temperature control. If the assay temperature fluctuates the results will be unreliable. In specialist laboratories, coagulation studies are undertaken on special apparatus, i.e. Coagulometer (Sarstedt).

INTERPRETATION OF HAEMATOLOGICAL VARIATIONS

The interpretation of haematological results is probably one of the most difficult aspects of the subject and there are certain rules which must be observed if full diagnostic value is to be obtained.

1. It is essential that a complete clinical examination has been undertaken prior to the haematological tests and that the haematological results are related to the clinical signs shown by the patient.
2. The practitioner has knowledge of normal haematological values and is aware of normal physiological variations.
3. The practitioner is aware of the type of haematological change which may occur in various pathological processes.
4. A single haematological examination may not yield definite results, and a second examination may be necessary.

NORMAL VALUES

Table 5.2 gives normal values for adult dogs and cats plus a few of the more unusual pets a practitioner will encounter.

Normal Physiological variations

Under certain normal circumstances, the figures quoted for normal adults may not apply. For instance, puppies and kittens have low red cell counts at birth and the values remain below adult levels until the animals are about 4 months old. Oestrus and pregnancy have effects on the white cell picture with variable degrees of neutrophilia increasing the total counts. Animals which struggle during examination may also have raised packed cell volumes and total white cell counts. Hamsters during hibernation have raised packed cell volumes and very low total white cell counts.

Treatment Variations

As well as physiological variations, there are also variations introduced by treatment which distort the picture. Treatment with corticosteroids is a widespread form of therapy and it produces marked neutrophilia and leucocytosis in most species. The degree of change depends on the dose and duration of treatment, but it is safe to assume that interpretation of white cell counts is often difficult when the patient is on corticosteroid therapy.

Table 5.2
Normal Adult Haematological Values

Species	R.B.C. x10^{12}/l	P.V.C. l/l	Hb. g/dl	W.B.C. x 10^9/l	Neutro-phils x 10^9/l	Lympho-cytes x 10^9/l	Mono-cytes x 10^9/l	Eosino-phils x 10^9/l	Baso-phils x 10^9/l
Dog	5.5-8.5* (6.4)	0.37-0.55* (0.45)	12.0-18.0* (15.0)	6.0-15.0 (10.1)	3.6-11.5 (6.3)	0.72-4.8 2.5)	0.18-1.5 (0.53)	0.12-1.5 (0.7)	0-0.1
Cat	5.5-10.0 (7.5)	0.24-0.45 (0.37)	8.0-14.0 (12.0)	7.0-20.0 (12.5)	2.5-12.5 (7.4)	1.5-7.0 (4.0)	0-0.85 (0.35)	0-1.5 (0.65)	0-0.1
Rabbit	4.0-7.0 (6.0)	0.30-0.50 (0.40)	8.0-15.0 (12.0)	6.0-12.0 (9.0)	2.0-6.0 (4.0)	2.0-5.0 (3.6)	0.1-1.0 (0.6)	0-0.5 (0.2)	0-1.0 (0.5)
Mouse	7.0-11.0 (9.0)	0.35-0.45 (0.40)	10.0-20.0 (15.0	4.0-12.0 (8.0	0.5-4.0 (1.8)	3.0-9.0 (5.45)	0-1.0 (0.5)	0-0.5 (0.2)	0-0.1 (0.05)
Guinea Pig	4.0-7.0 (6.0)	0.35-0.45 (0.40)	11.0-17.0 (14.0)	7.0-14.0 (10.0)	2.0-6.0 (4.0)	3.0-8.0 (5.0)	0.2-2.0 (0.5)	0-2.0 (0.5)	0-0.5 (0.1)
Golden Hamster	6.0-9.0 (7.0)	0.42-0.53 (0.48)	14.0-19.0 (16.0)	5.0-10.0 (7.0)	1.0-4.0 (2.03)	3.5-8.0 (4.76)	0.07-0.5 (0.14)	0-0.25 (0.07)	Rare

N.B. Figures in brackets represent averages.

* *Figures are higher for some breeds, notably the greyhound*

Surgical intervention also results in leucocytosis and haematology is of limited diagnostic value in animals which have had recent surgery.

It is worth remembering that laboratory results have to be interpreted with great caution when the patient has been receiving therapy prior to the samples being taken.

ABNORMAL HAEMATOLOGICAL VARIATIONS

It is more realistic to consider all the estimations relating to red cells or white cells as one diagnostic unit, rather than considering each estimation as an isolated entity. In practice, consideration of all the haematological results at the same time is a desirable target, but, for the purposes of this section it is more convenient and explicit if they are considered in three groups: red cells, white cells and clotting defects.

Red cell indices

The total red cell count may be above or below normal and the packed cell volume and haemoglobin values will follow the total counts. **Increased** values are generally associated with dehydration and should be interpreted only after appraisal of the patient's clinical condition. Often, the red cell indices rise only when dehydration is advanced. **Reduced** red cell values indicate anaemia, but the interpretation of the results is complicated. To know an animal is anaemic is a useful observation but to know exactly **why** it is anaemic is even more useful. Achieving this second goal is not easy and may often prove to be impossible. Establishing the cause of anaemia entails looking at the values for total red cell count, packed cell volume and haemoglobin. From these, one can deduce how severe the anaemia is. You then have to find out if the anaemia is present because the animal has lost more blood than the bone marrow can replace, or whether the anaemia is caused by bone marrow failure. The history and clinical signs may help here, i.e. history of haemorrhage.

Laboratory evidence is increased by undertaking reticulocyte counts (excessive numbers indicate the bone marrow is functioning rapidly), by estimating corpuscular values and by studying a stained smear for evidence of erythrocyte regeneration, i.e. polychromasia, occurrence of large immature cells, etc.

If evidence suggests anaemia and there is no sign of excessive red cell regeneration, then the bone marrow may be faulty due to a variety of causes such as malnutrition, severe parasitism, terminal effects of neoplasia, etc. Remember that the bone marrow may take a day or two following acute haemorrhage to show signs of hyper-activity. Do not confuse this delay with anaemia due to bone marrow failure. If signs of marrow activity are obvious, then the anaemia must be due to haemorrhage or haemolysis. Haemorrhage, including bleeding into the gut, is usually detectable clinically. Internal haemorrhage can be suspected from the clinical history. Haemolysis may be less easy to detect clinically unless jaundice appears. Once the possible cause is identified, i.e. haemorrhage, then further steps should be taken to find out exactly where the bleeding is coming from and why, i.e. is the clotting mechanism efficient, is this a localised source of blood loss such as an ulcer, etc?

Haematology is used to try to establish if anaemia is present. How severe it is, whether the animal is producing new cells and, later, to try to define precisely the cause. Repeat samples are useful to establish if the anaemia has been overcome and, if so, how effectively.

White cell indices

These are more complicated, change in a less specific manner than red cells and the results are, consequently, less easy to interpret. The results of total and differential white cell counts are used, in the main, to detect disease trends rather than pinpoint specific diseases. In general, it should be assumed that total and differential white cell counts are screening tests used to detect pathological changes, such as inflammation or neoplasia.

Explanation of various types of white cell change.
  i. Neutrophils help to combat inflammation.
  ii. Immature neutrophils are produced when the demand for neutrophils outstrips the supply (shift to the left).
  iii. If immature neutrophil numbers are raised but mature neurophils predominate, this is a regenerative shift to the left indicating that the body defences are active.
  iv. If immature neutrophil numbers exceed mature neutrophils (degenerative shift to the left) this indicates that the inflammation is overwhelming the body defences.
  v. Total circulating neutrophil numbers are not always directly related to the severity of the illness, but in general, particularly in the dog and cat, the higher the neutrophil numbers the more acute and severe is the clinical illness.
  vi. Lymphocytes are concerned with immune defence mechanisms.
  vii. Increasing lymphocyte numbers may indicate an excessive antibody defence reaction or it may be due to neoplasia of lymphocytes.
  viii. Decreased lymphocyte numbers are associated with shock or stress of variable origin.
  ix. Persistently low lymphocyte numbers indicate a poor prognosis.
  x. Eosinophils respond to the presence of histamine and circulating numbers increase, particularly in allergies and parasitism. Low eosinophil numbers are associated with stress of variable origin, although eosinophil numbers may be low in perfectly healthy animals.
  xi. Monocytes are involved in the removal of tissue debris and hence they are particularly numerous in chronic disease when debris builds up. Their numbers are a reflection of disease duration.

  The total white cell count may be above, within or below the normal range during a disease process and the differential count may vary within each category.

Total white cell count above normal
Interpretation of this type of result will depend on how high the total count is and what cell types are involved. The higher the total count, the more serious the process which stimulated the leucocytosis. It is absolutely essential to correlate the total and differential counts, otherwise serious mistakes can be made. If, for example, the total count is 20.0 x 10^9/l and the neutrophils percentage is 50, this is equivalent to 10.0 x 10^9/l neutrophils. If the total count is 50.0 x 10^9/l and the neutrophils account for 70% of the total, this is equivalent to 35.0 x 10^9/l and the interpretation would be different. Always try to gauge leucocyte changes by using absolute figures rather than percentages and comparing them with the normal range for absolute figures.

Neutrophils. Increasing absolute numbers of neutrophils indicate inflammation and the greater degree of shift to the left, the more acute and severe the condition. Total white cell counts may increase due to neutro philia and, in general terms, total counts of 15.0—25.0 x 10^9/l indicate moderate inflammatory reactions, and counts of between 25.0 and 35.0 x 10^9/l indicate more severe reactions in the dog. Total counts in excess of 35.0 x 10^9/l should be viewed with concern. These figures need some adjustment in the cat, a species with a normally high total white cell count (Table 5.2).

If the total counts reach 100.0 x 10^9/l then neoplasia should be considered seriously, although non-tumourous inflammation can stimulate such high counts on occasion. The interpretation of leucocytosis due to neutrophilia can only be made when the following factors are taken into consideration.

    i. Total white blood cell count.

    ii Number of mature and immature neutrophils.

    iii. Duration and type of clinical illness.

    iv. Species of animal.

All four have a bearing on the final interpretation and simple explanations are not available, although the following may be an interpretation guide.

a.   The higher the total count with neutrophilia and shift to the left, the more severe the condition.

b.   Moderate total counts with many immature neutrophils indicate poor prognosis.

c.   Acute foci of inflammation stimulate greater neutrophil responses.

d.   Inflammation sites which are draining (open abscesses, open pyrometra) stimulate only moderate neutrophilia.

e.   Chronic, walled-off lesions, even when extensive, stimulate little neutrophil response.

Lymphocytes. The normal lymphocyte numbers vary markedly in the species listed in table 5.2. In these species, with normally high lymphocyte counts, i.e. mice, slight alteration in percentages following immune responses will go unnoticed. In the dog and cat, immunology stimulated increases may be more apparent but it would be very unusual if they increased to an extent which would raise the lymphocyte figures above 10.0 x 10^9/l. In neoplastic conditions (lymphosarcoma) absolute lymphocyte numbers may increase markedly and exceed 100.0 x 10^9/l, but in many cases increases are moderate or imperceptible and lymphocyte morphology is a surer, but not infallible, way of confirming a tentative diagnosis. In general terms, haematology will confirm lymphosarcoma only in those cases showing marked deviation in the number and type of lymphocytes. In the majority of cases haematology is of little or no diagnostic assistance in the early stages of the disease even if lymph node enlargement is apparent.

Monocytes. Absolute monocyte numbers increase in chronic diseases, especially those in which excess tissue debris accumulates. In the dog and cat the increases are limited and only in exceptional cases will the total number of monocytes exceed 5.0 x 10^9/l, so that their effect on total leucocyte numbers is restricted. Monocyte numbers do not reveal the precise cause of the illness.

Eosinophils. Variation in circulating eosinophil numbers is transient and can easily be missed. Numbers increase, although they rarely exceed 4.0 x 10^9/l in the dog and cat, in cases of allergy, parasitism and chronic skin dieases of varying aetiology. If eosinophil numbers are significantly raised and one of the aforementioned clinical entities is suspected, the test is useful. Massive increases in eosinophil numbers are occasionally seen in dogs and cats with neoplasia, especially lymphosarcoma. In such cases the eosinophil percentage may exceed 50 and in absolute terms, values above 10 x 10^9/l can be seen. Negative findings with regard to raised eosinophil numbers do not mean that the conditions are absent.

Total white cell count below normal
Basically, there are four sets of conditions which can lead to a reduced total white cell count.

i.   Bone marrow failure.

ii   Overwhelming infections.

iii   Viral diseases.

iv.   Other disorders.

Bone marrow failure. This is unusual and the reduced white cell total would be accompanied by reduced red cell and platelet counts and there would be no evidence of active cellular regeneration when the blood smears were examined. The most likely causes are severe malnutrition and cachexia following prolonged disease processes.

Overwhelming infections. In this case, the total white cell count may be normal or slightly below normal. There will evidence of a disproportionately large percentage of immature neutrophils and reduced levels of mature neutrophils, lymphocytes and eosinophils. In such cases the prognosis without treatment is poor.

Viral infections. Many viral infections have the effect of depressing the number of circulating leucocytes, especially neutrophils and lymphocytes. In many of these infections the initial viral effects are rapidly superseded by bacterial secondaries and the bone marrow responds to these pathogens by neutrophilia, often resulting in leucocytosis. In these instances, by the time the animal is presented for examination, the initial viral changes have disappeared. This type of pattern occurs in diseases such as distemper and upper respiratory infections. In infectious feline panleucopenia, this pattern is not followed. The viral effects are severe and prolonged, including a marked leucopenia with total white cell counts below $2.0 \times 10^9/l$ and often as low as $0.5 \times 10^9/l$. Neutrophil and lymphocyte numbers are drastically reduced. This type of blood picture, taken in conjunction with the clinical signs, can be diagnostic. Canine parvovirus produces similar severe leucocyte depletion, but the effects do not last as long and it is possible to see early clinical cases in which the leucopenia is being superseded by neutrophilia.

On occasion, individual cell types may be reduced in number but in most cases this reduction does not lower the total count appreciably. For example, lymphocyte and eosinophil numbers decline in conditions of stress, but this change is usually compensated for by raised neutrophil counts and the total white cell count may, in fact, rise.

Other conditions. There are some conditions, often of an endocrinological nature which preferentially reduce the numbers of certain cells, e.g. Cushing's disease induces a fall in the eosinophil count and may remove eosinophils completely.

Clotting defects

These are unusual but, when they do occur, haematological assistance can be of great value. The rarer conditions, such as haemophilia, need sophisticated laboratory techniques for specific confirmation but the activated partial thromboplastin test will act as a guide. Those conditions which are seen more often and require relatively simple laboratory tests for confirmation, include Warfarin poisoning and thrombocytopenia.

Warfarin poisoning can be confirmed if the clinical signs and history are suggestive, by estimating prothrombin time. The results will show a greatly extended time for a clot to form. In normal dogs, the prothrombin time is less than 20 seconds. In Warfarin poisoning (or prothrombinaemia due to liver failure) the time will exceed 30 seconds and, in most cases, be longer than 60 seconds.

Thrombocytopenia (platelet deficiency) is, in most cases, an acquired auto-immune phenomenon. The normal platelet count is all species is between $200.0 \times 10^9/l$ and $600.0 \times 10^9/l$. When bleeding occurs due to platelet deficiency, the number will be less than $20.0 \times 10^9/l$. Such a finding can be diagnostic, although additional tests such as a direct Coomb's test, will help to confirm a diagnosis. Platelet numbers may fall to levels of around $50.0 \times 10^9/l$ in animals with severe chronic haemorrhage unassociated with thrombocytopenia due solely to excessive demand for platelets.

OTHER INFORMATION

The values in this chapter are given in Système Internationale d.Unités (SI Units) which may not be familiar. Below are examples of the old and new recording units.

	OLD UNITS	SI UNITS
Total red cell count	millions/cu.mm. (e.g. 5,000,000 per cu.mm.	$\times 10_{12}$/litre = 5.0×10^{12}/l)
Total white cell count	thousands/cu.mm. (e.g. 5,000 per cu.mm.	$\times 10^9$/l) = 5.0×10^9/l)
Packed cell volume	percentage (e.g. 45%	litre/litre = 0.45 l/l)
Haemoglobin	grams/100 mls (e.g. 15.0 g/100 ml	grams/decilitre = 15.0 g/dl)
Mean cell volume*	$c\mu$	femto litres (fl)
Mean cell haemoglobin	$\mu\mu$g	picograms (pg)
Mean cell haemoglobin concentration	percentage	grams/decilitre

*Corpuscular values — only a change in nomenclature — i.e. 70.0 $c\mu$ = 70.0 fl

FURTHER READING

Acevedo R.A. *et al.,* 1981. Am. J. vet. Res.**42**: 537

Jahanmehr, S.A.H., Hyde, K., Gleary, C.G., Cinkotal, K.I., and MacIver, J.E. J. Clin. Path. **40,** 1987, 926—929

Schalm's Veterinary Haematology. Jain, N.C. 4th edition 1986. Lea and Febiger, Philadelphia.

CHAPTER 6

EXTERNAL PARASITES

G. S. Walton B.V.Sc., M.R.C.V.S.

INTRODUCTION

The presence of ectoparasitic infestations of the dog and cat may often be suspected in the clinical case after carrying out a careful macroscopical examination of the presenting pattern of cutaneous change.

Confirmation of diagnosis can only be achieved following the collection and subsequent identification of the relevant parasite by laboratory examination of suitable material or skin samples.

SAMPLING TECHNIQUES

SAMPLE COLLECTION

1. **Direct Isolation and Removal of Ectoparasites**

   Apparatus: Suitable source of illumination, hand lens or illumination map reading glass, forceps, swab sticks, dissecting needles, parasiticidal aerosol spray, quill fashion comb or fine toothed metal comb, large sheet of plastic or paper, aspirator.

   Techniques: Search coat using comb or fingers to turn back hair. On sighting ectoparasites either with the naked eye or aided by a hand lens or map reading glass, remove parasite either manually or with an aspirator (fleas), forceps (lice and lice eggs), moistened swab stick or dissecting needles (cheyletiella, forage mites, harvest mites, otodectes).

   Advantages: Rapid method for heavy infestations (lice, cheyletiella, otodectes, harvest mite and larger species of forage mites).

   Disadvantages: Difficult and laborious in light infestations. Recovery of fleas may be improved by prior use of a suitable parasiticidal aerosol or by placing the body of the animal in a large plastic bag immediately after it has been destroyed and then either using a parasiticide or refrigeration.

2. **General Body Grooming**

   Apparatus: Quill fashion comb or fine toothed metal comb, large sheet of plastic or paper, parasiticidal aerosol spray.

   Technique: Place subject on large sheet of plastic or paper. Apply adequate restraint. Groom thoroughly and collect all debris that falls onto sheeting. In suspected flea infestations, spray subject with suitable parasiticidal aerosol spray prior to grooming.

   Advantages: Rapid. Valuable in cases of low infestation and for the collection of flea debris.

   Disadvantages: Necessary to separate skin debris from hair, grit and sand manually prior to laboratory examination.

3. Collection using Quill Fashion Comb

Apparatus: Quill Fashion Comb, large sheet of plastic or paper.

Technique: Restrain subject. Examine thoroughly. Select suitable area of hyperaemia and scaling. Position over sheeting. Scrub area using comb. Collect skin debris from sheeting.

Advantages: Rapid. Possible to collect large amounts of material. No danger of injury to patient. No clipping of hair required in the majority of cases. Valuable for the detection of sarcoptes, notoedres, forage mites, harvest mites, cheyletiella and demodex mites.

Disadvantages: Necessary to separate skin debris from hair, grit and sand manually prior to laboratory examination.

4. Collection of Material using Sellotape

Apparatus: Sellotape, scissors or clippers, microscope slide.

Technique: Select area of scaling and hyperaemia. Remove hair. Press tape firmly onto skin and then remove and mount on microscope slide with or without KOH.

Advantages: Rapid. Valuable as a research method and for the diagnosis of cheyletiella and, on occasions, demodex infestations.

Disadvantages: Only possible to collect a limited amount of material. Mites may be obscured by debris. Unsatisfactory for sarcoptes diagnosis. Necessary to denude of hair.

5. Collection of Hair by Skin Scraping

Apparatus: Scalpel blade, scissors, microscopic slides, light lubricating oil or 10% KOH.

Technique: Select area of hyperaemia and scaling. Clip away hair. Pinch up skin into fold. Moisten with a drop of oil or KOH. Scrape skin several times in one direction. Wipe scale which collects on blade onto microscope slide. Repeat process until bleeding noted.

Advantages: Possible to take deep skin samples. When oil is used, specimens remain fresh for several days.

Disadvantages: Area denuded. Danger if patient moves. Time consuming when large amount of material is required. Impossible to clear specimens when oil is used. Mites may be mutilated during collection.

6. Collection of Material from Pustules

Apparatus: Microscope slide.

Technique: Select pustule. Squeeze contents onto microscope slide.

Advantages: Very rapid method of diagnosis of demodex infestation when pustules present.

Disadvantages: Only of advantage in demodex infestations.

7. Collection of Material from Habitat

Apparatus: Vacuum cleaner, large sheet of plastic or paper.

Technique: Material may be collected from flooring using vacuum cleaners. Blankets should be shaken over sheeting and debris collected.

Advantages: Valuable for assessing infestation of environment in flea infestations. Often essential in Dermannysus infestations.

Disadvantages: Laboratory examination of material time consuming.

8. Biopsy Material

Apparatus: Dental syringe, Keyes punch (4 mm), forceps, 10% Formol saline, scissors, surgical spirit.

Technique: Clip away hair. Clean site with surgical spirit, remove plug of skin using punch and place material in fixative.

Advantages: Occasionally of value in demodex infestations.

Disadvantages: Expensive, time consuming. Unreliable for other ectoparasitic infestations, including sarcoptes and notoedres, even after performing serial sectioning of biopsy material.

9. **Faecal Material**

   Apparatus: Spatula, faeces pots.

   Technique: Straightforward.

   Advantages: Mites often found on routine examination of material.

   Disadvantages: Infestations may require examination of large amounts of faecal material before positive diagnosis achieved.

SAMPLE TRANSPORT

1. **Sealed plastic bags**

   Comment: Essential to remove air before sealing. Samples remain in satisfactory condition for several days, providing not obtained from suppurating lesions or subject to prior moistening with either water or KOH.

2. **In mineral oils**

   Comment: Keep well for several days. Very difficult to clear material should this be required during subsequent laboratory examination.

3. **In Surgical Spirit (70% Ethyl Alcohol)**

   Comment: Shrinkage of mites may occur.

4. **Oudeman's Solution**
   Formulation: Ethyl alcohol (70%)   87 parts
   Glycerine   5 parts
   Glacial acetic acid   8 parts

   Comments: Valuable for short term preservation of mites, but not all larger ectoparasites.

LABORATORY METHODS

MOUNTING FLUIDS

1. **Water**

   Use only when nothing else available. Unsatisfactory when clearing or preservation of preparation required.

2. **Glycerine and Glycerine Jelly**

   Useful temporary mount, when clearing of preparation not required.

3. **Potassium Hydroxide (10 or 20%)**

   Useful for initial examination. Possible to clear specimens either by heating **gently** or leaving overnight in a moist chamber.

4. **Light Lubricating Oil**

   Useful when no clearing of preparation required. Will preserve parasite for several days.

5. **Lactic Acid**

Will clear preparations when warmed gently. Only useful as temporary mountant.

6. **Lactophenol**

Formulation: Phenol   20g
                Lactic acid   16.5 ml
                Glycerol   32.0 ml
                Dist. water   20.0 ml

Helpful for clearing specimens, can cause shrinkage of soft bodied mites.

7. **C. M. Mounting Media**

Formulation: Methocellulose   5g.
                Ethyl alcohol (95%) 25ml
                Carbowax   2g
                Diethylglycol   1 ml
                Lactic acid   100 ml
                Distilled water   75 ml

Mix methocellulose and alcohol. Add remainder. Filter through glass wool. Mature by incubating for 5 days at 40°C. Little shrinkage. Preserves specimens for several years.

EXAMINATION TECHNIQUES

1. **Direct examination using Dissection Microscope**

Apparatus: Plastic petri dishes, dissecting needles, warming plate (45°C).

Technique: Place debris to be examined in petri dish. Leave 12−24 hours then transfer petri dish and contents onto warming plate for 10 minutes. Observe under microscope for movement and subsequent identification of mites.

Advantages: Useful for the examination of skin debris and vacuumings from animal houses. Can be used for identification of lice and larger ectoparasites.

Disadvantages: Little value for detection of parasites in old samples.

2. **Direct Microscopic Examination**

Apparatus: Plain or hollowed microscopic slides, coverslips, dissecting needles, mounting fluid, microscope, source of heat.

Technique: Place selected ectoparasite together with drop of mounting fluid on either a plain or hollowed microscope slide. Examine under low power objective. Reposition if required (customery to mount fleas right side down). Gently lower coverslip onto preparation.

Samples of scale and debris may be mounted on a microscope slide with either KOH or lactic acid and covered with either a second slide or a coverslip after spreading the material evenly over the low slide. Gently warm or leave the preparation to clear. Adjust the microscope sub-stage condenser and diaphragm to provide an evenly distributed, but relatively low intensity of light. Scan the material on the slide methodically. This may be followed by a more detailed study of an individual ectoparasite under higher power if a coverslip has been used during preparation.

Advantages: Routine method of study of individually mounted ectoparasites. Rapid method for routine screening of small amounts of skin debris or scrapings.

Disadvantages: There may be some difficulty in clearing material containing heavily pigmented epithelial debris adequately. Time consuming if large amounts of skin debris require examination.

3. **Examination following Sedimentation**

Apparatus: Test-tube, 10% KOH, source of heat, pipette, centrifuge, slides, coverslips.

Technique: Place skin debris or scrapings into test tube. Boil gently until all debris has dissolved.

Allow sedimentation or spin down. Pipette off supernatant fluid. Use deposit to make smears. Subject to direct microscopical examination.

Advantages: Valuable when larger amount of material requires examination.

Disadvantages: Ectoparasites may be damaged or destroyed if boiled excessively. Still time consuming. Not satisfactory for permanent mounting.

4. **Sugar flotation modification**

   Apparatus: As for (3), plus saturated sugar solution.

   Technique: As for (3), but after removal of supernatant, half fill test-tube with water and then complete filling using saturated sugar solution. Centrifuge (1000 r.p.m.) for one minute. Remove parasites from the surface film using a slide or cover slip. Subject to direct microscopical examination.

   Advantages: Valuable for screening large amounts of material and the diagnosis of mite infestations.

   Disadvantages: Difficult to make satisfactory permanent mounts.

INTERPRETATION OF RESULTS

IDENTIFICATION OF ECTOPARASITES

Fleas

The shape and approximate size of the common ectoparasites is shown in Figure 6.1.

Faecal material: Black gritty specks, which, on dissolving in water or KOH, appear as cherry red homogenous masses, devoid of fibrin crystals or epithetial tissue.

Larva: White segmented, occasionally found in pelt of long coated animals and bedding.

Eggs: Small white oval, occasionally found in coat or bedding.

Adults: Reddish brown, laterally compressed, hard shiny bodied, prominent legs, head fused into thorax, capable of rapid movement and jumping. Species identification complex, requiring detailed examination and expert knowledge.

Comment: Confirmation of diagnosis can be difficult in cases of flea hypersensitivity, when severe skin changes may be produced during or following low grade or intermittent flea infestation.

Lice

Eggs: Cemented directly to hair, white, oval with cupola.

Adults: *Trichodectes canis* (Dog and Cat), *Filicola subrostratus* (Cat) biting lice, soft bodied, 1.0—1.9 mm long, grey soft bodied, flattened dorso-ventrally with domed head wider than thorax. *Linognathus setosus* (Cat), sucking louse, soft grey body, elongated head narrower than thorax.

Comment: Direct isolation often requires careful and prolonged scanning of the coat, as parasite numbers can be very low and confined to specific areas of the body (the flaps of long eared dogs or discrete areas of the trunk in other dog breeds and cats).

Sarcoptes

Eggs: Non-attached, oval.

Adults: Oval, 0.2—0.4 mm long, terminal anus, short legs, suckers on legs 1 and 2 (female), 1, 2 and 4 (male).

Comment: In the dog, infestation is frequently confined to the face, edges of the ear flap, ventral chest and limbs. In large breeds, the face and ears can be spared. Infestation may involve the trunk

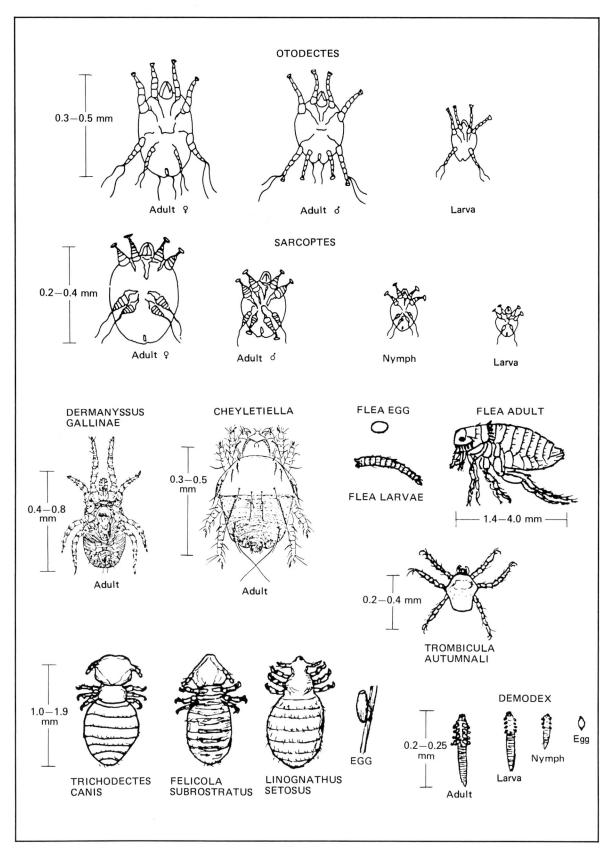

Figure 6.1

in the puppy. As mite numbers are frequently low, large amounts of material may need to be examined before diagnosis can be confirmed; careful selection of the site from which the material is collected is essential. The identification of either a single mite or embryonated egg is diagnostic.

Notoedres

Comment: Material should be collected from areas of scaling and inflammation usually involving the head, neck or trunk. Confirmation of diagnosis as for sarcoptes.

Otodectes

Eggs: Non-attached, oval.

Adults: Oval shaped body 0.3—0.5 mm long, long legs, with suckers on legs 1 and 2 (female), 1, 2, 3 and 4 (male).

Comment: Severity of ear inflammation is not correlated to mite numbers.

Cheyletiella

Eggs: Non-attached, oval.

Adults: Shield shaped body, 0.3—0.5 mm long. Terminal combs instead of suckers on legs. Prominent accessory mouth parts (palpi) terminating in well developed curved hooks. Species identification of sensory organ shape situated on 1st leg and minor anatomical differences.

Comment: Skin responses associated with this parasite very variable; many animals appearing clinically normal, with little evidence of irritation or skin change despite severe responses being noted in individual animal and human contacts.

Trombicula Autumnali

Larva: Red oval body 0.2—0.4 mm, 3 pairs of long legs each terminating in three hooks (middle hook longer than others).

Comment: Larva have distinct geographical distribution and pronounced seasonal activity. Areas of focal infestation often observed involving the legs, lower trunk and/or face.

Forage mites

Morphology: Extremely variable in size and shape. Identification of individual members of this very large group requires detailed examination and considerable expertise.

Demodex

Eggs: Small oval packets.

Larva: Cigar shaped with three pairs of legs anteriorly.

Nymph: Cigar shaped, four pairs of legs anteriorly.

Adult: Cigar shaped, 0.2—0.25 mm long, four pairs of legs anteriorly.

Dermannysus Gallinae and other bird mites

Comment: Many fowl mites are nocturnal feeders, leaving their 'hosts' during the day and hiding in bedding, floor, wall or ceiling crevices.

ADDITIONAL INFORMATION

FURTHER READING

EVANS, G. O. J., SHEALS, E. G. AND MACFARLANE, D. (1961). *The Terrestrial Acari of the British Isles:* An Introduction to their Morphology, Biology and Classification. The Trustees of the British Museum, London.

FLYNN, R. J. (1973). *Parasites of Laboratory Animals.* Iowa State University Press. Ames, Iowa.

HOPKINS G. H. E. and ROTHSCHILD, M. (1953). *An illustrated Catalogue of the Rothschild Collection of Fleas (Siphonaptera) in the British Museum (Natural History).* Vol 1. Tungidae and Pulicidae. The Trustees of the British Museum, London.

HUGHES, A. M. (1961). *Mites of Stored Food.* (Technical Bulletin No. 9 M.A.F.F.) H.M.S.C.

MULLER, G. H., KIRK, R. W. and SCOTT, D. W. (1983) *Small Animal Dermatology.* 3rd Ed. W. B. Saunders, Philadelphia.

SLOSS, M. W. and KEMP, R. L. (1978) *Veterinary Clinical Parasitology.* Iowa State University Press, Ames, Iowa.

SMIT, F. G. A. M. (1954). *Handbook for the Identification of Insects of Medical Importance.* 2nd Ed. The Trustees of the British Museum, London.

CHAPTER 7

INTERNAL PARASITES

J. Armour Ph.D., Dr.h.c.(Utrecht), M.R.C.V.S.

INTRODUCTION

The presence of mature helminth or protozoal infections in the alimentary and respiratory tracts of pet animals can often be detected microscopically by the appearance of the appropriate eggs or larval stages in the faeces. On gross examination of faeces, tapeworm segments are often seen and, during the summer, larvae of various dipterin flies may also occur *(Paregle radicum)*. In certain of the respiratory tract infections the examination of sputum for larvae may also prove beneficial. Some species of nematode larvae and protozoa also occur in blood and may be detected by examination of stained or lysed blood smears. Techniques for detection of internal parasite infections are outlined below.

SAMPLE COLLECTION

Faecal samples should always be fresh and preferably collected directly from the rectum using a plastic finger stall or a plastic glove. Alternatively, the sample can be collected as it is passed. For small pets a thermometer or glass rod may be used. The collection of samples from the ground is sometimes unavoidable but there is always a risk of contamination with free living nematodes. Ideally, at least 5 g of faeces should be collected since this amount is required for some of the concentration methods of examination.

Since eggs embryonate rapidly the faeces should be stored in the refrigerator unless examination is carried out within a day. For samples sent through the post, the addition of twice the faecal volume of 10% formalin to the faeces will minimise development and hatching. Blood samples should be collected in EDTA or in citrate for clotting times (see page 56).

The collection of tracheal sputum with the end of a bronchoscope is often the best method of collecting the larvae of *Oslerus (Filaroides) osleri* or *Filaroides hirthi.* If a bronchoscope is not available then direct collections of sputum from the pharyngeal area should be attempted.

LABORATORY METHODS

ROUTINE FAECES EXAMINATION

1. **Direct Smear Method**

   Apparatus: Slides, coverslips and microscope.
   Technique: Place a few drops of water on a slide. Mix a little faeces into water with scalpel blade or matchstick.
   Attach coverslip and examine microscopically. Screen under X25 objective.

   Advantages: Ease of preparation, not costly.
   Disadvantages: Purely qualitative. Detects only heavy infections. Differentation of small eggs such as oocysts is difficult.

2.   Flotation Methods

Apparatus: Slides, coverslips (22 mm square), 15 ml flat bottomed test tubes, tea strainer, bowl and microscope. If available, centrifuge with swing-out head.

Solutions: Flotation solutions are used at saturation or near saturation. Use either.

Saturated salt	Sp. gr. 1.2
Zinc sulphate	Sp. gr. 1.33
Magnesium sulphate	Sp. gr. 1.35
Sugar	Sp. gr. 1.35

Technique: Without centrifugation.

Mix 3 or 4 gms of faeces with 50 ml water. Pour mixture through 100 mesh sieve (a tea strainer will do) into a bowl.
Rotate bowl and tip filtrate into two test tubes and allow to sediment for 5 minutes.
Remove supernatant and mix sediment with enough flotation solution to ensure a positive meniscus at top of the tube.
Place coverslips on tubes and allow to stand for 15 minutes.
Remove coverslips from each tube in one motion and examine microscopically.
Use X25 objective to screen for helminth eggs; for coccidia oocysts or larvae a higher magnification is better.

Technique: With centrifugation.

As above except that both the faeces suspension in water and subsequently in flotation fluid should be spun at 1500 r.p.m. for 3 minutes in lieu of standing period. Some laboratories apply the coverslip prior to second centrifugation but care must be taken that a good contact exists between coverslip and test tube.

Advantages: Clear preparation (particularly if centrifuged).

Disadvantages: Qualitative.

3.   Modified McMaster Method

Apparatus: Balance, beakers, 15 ml flat-bottomed test tubes, strainer, bowl, centrifuge, Pasteur pipettes, microscope and McMaster slides.

Solutions: Saturated salt is most common.

Technique: Thoroughly mix 3 gms of faeces with 42 ml of water (a mechanical stirrer is an advantage). Pour mixture through 100 mesh sieve or strainer into bowl.
Tip filtrate into a 15 ml test tube and centrifuge for 3 minutes at 1500 r.p.m. Discard supernatant, agitate sediment and fill test tube with salt solution.
Invert tube 6 or 7 times keeping thumb over the end and withdraw sufficient fluid into Pasteur pipette to fill one chamber of the McMaster slide (0.15 ml).
Repeat and fill other chamber (N.B. It helps to wet the slide prior to filling).
Examine McMaster slide (Figure 7.1) using the X4 objective of the microscope. Count the total eggs within lined areas of both chambers. The number of eggs per gm is obtained by multiplying the total number of eggs by 50. (3 gm of faeces gave 45 ml suspension and 2 x 0.15 ml, i.e. 0.3 ml are examined).

Advantages: Quantitative.

Disadvantages: More costly. Detailed identification of smaller eggs, such as coccidia oocysts or larvae is difficult.

SPECIAL TECHNIQUES

1.   Simple Baermann Method (for recovery of larvae from faeces.)

Apparatus: Beaker, muslin, test tubes, Pasteur pipettes, coverslips and slides.
Technique: Take 10 gms of faeces and wrap in muslin. Suspend muslin bag containing faeces in a beaker of warm water and leave overnight (see Figure 7.2).

Syphon or pour off most of supernatant and pour remaining sediment into test tube.
Allow to stand for 2 hours and pour off supernatant.
Add a few drops of clean water to sediment, agitate and pipette on to slides. Place coverslips on top and examine with X40 or X100 objective.

Advantages: Detects low numbers of first stage larvae of *O. osleri, Angiostronglylus, Aelurostrongylus vasorum* or *A. abstrusus*.

2. Modified Baermann Method

Apparatus: Filter paper (17 cm.), retort stand, filter funnel, rubber tubing and clip, sieve, beaker, test tubes, slides, coverslips and microscope.

Technique: Spread 10 gms. of faeces thinly on 17 cm filter paper.
Place sieve in contact with warm water in funnel with rubber hose and clip (see Figure 7.2).
Reverse filter paper and place on sieve.
Leave overnight.
Release clip and run off water from bottom of funnel into beaker.
Pour into test tube and allow to sediment.
Remove supernatant and screen sediment on slides under x40 objective.
If larvae are present use X100 objective for species identification.

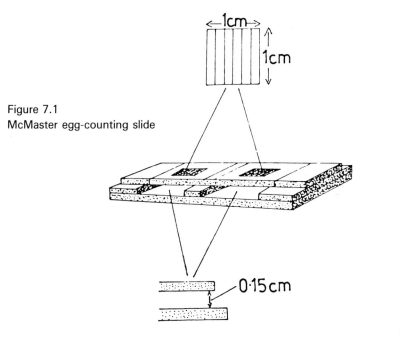

Figure 7.1
McMaster egg-counting slide

Figure 7.2
Baermann apparatus

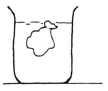

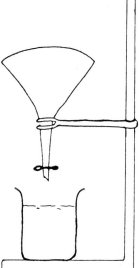

OTHER AIDS TO DIAGNOSIS

Blood examination

Routine blood techniques such as red cell counts, haemoglobin estimation and calculation of the packed cell volume percentages will indicate the presence of anaemia. Mild anaemia may occur in several intestinal infections such as *Uncinaria* and *Toxocara* or *Trichuris* and *Isospora* infections in indigenous dogs and *Ancylostoma* in imported dogs.

Several blood parasites may also occur, particularly in imported animals, including the nematode filarioids *Dirofilaria immitis* and *Dipetalonema reconditum* in dogs; the protozoa *Babesia canis* and *Trypanosoma brucei* in dogs and *Haemobartonella* spp. in dogs and cats. The presence of these parasites is best confirmed by blood smear, and reference should be made to a protozoology textbook for their morphology.

Two techniques are widely used for detection of blood parasites:

1. **Whole Blood Smear Stained by Giemsa.**

   Apparatus: Methyl alcohol, distilled water, slides, glass cylinder, microscope with oil immersion lens.

   Solution: Giemsa stain.

   Technique: Make the blood smear on two slides and dry in air.
   Fix in methyl alcohol for 3 minutes. Add ten drops of Giemsa stain to 10 ml of distilled water in cylinder.
   Pour over 2 slides and leave for 30 minutes.
   Rinse in distilled water for 10 minutes.
   Blot dry.
   Examine under oil immersion.

   Advantages: Detects both intracellular (*Babesia* spp., *Haemobartonella*) and extracellular parasites such as *Trypanosoma* and microfilariae of *Dirofilaria immitis* and *Dipetalonema reconditum.* Those of *D. immitis* are more than 300 µm in length and have a tapered head and a straight tail; those of *D. reconditum* are less than 300 µm and have a blunt head and a hooked posterior end. These measurements would require a measuring eyepiece and stage micrometer.

   Disadvantage: Does not detect low numbers of parasites.

2. **Lysed Blood Smear**

   Apparatus: Clean slides, conical test tubes, Pasteur pipette, microscope.

   Solutions: Methylene Blue, Formalin (2%).

   Technique: (Modified Knott's technique). Mix 1 ml of fresh blood with 9 ml of 2% formalin.
   Centrifuge for 8 minutes at 1500 r.p.m.
   Discard supernatant and mix sediment with an equal volume of 1:1000 methylene blue.
   Pipette on to slide and examine wet under x10 objective.

   Advantage: Detects low numbers of microfilariae which are easily measured.

   Disadvantage: Does not detect intracellular protozoa.

N.B. In areas where *Dirofilaria* is endemic, a special filtration technique has been developed and is available in kit form. These kits are not available in the U.K.*

*TILLEY, L.P. and WILKINS, R.J. The Difil Test Kit for detection of Canine Heartworm microfilaria. VM/SAC 69 (1974) 288.
WYLIE, J. P. Detection of microfilaria by a filter technique. JAVMA 156 (1970) 1403.

Blood Clotting Time (see also page 66).

Where *Angiostrongylus vasorum* infection in the dog is suspected, an estimation of blood clotting time is useful. The normal clotting time of dog's blood is 5—8 minutes. In dogs infected with *A. vasorum* it is in excess of 12 minutes.

Sputum Examination

The sputum should be mixed with a few drops of water and spread on a slide, covered with a coverslip and screened under the X25 objective. Final identification of *Oslerus osleri* can be made under X40.

Serological Examination

Confirmation of *Toxoplasma gondii* infection is normally made by serological examination. The Sabin-Feldman Dye Test is still used but only in a few specialised laboratories for confirmation of other test results. Several other tests are now available in specialised laboratories including the Indirect Fluorescence antibody technique and the indirect haemagglutination test. A few laboratories have an ELISA test available and there is a commercially available: Japanese latex agglutination test (Eiken Chemical Co. Ltd). In cats, a 1:32 titre is doubtful and a 1:64 titre positive with latex agglutination. Ideally, for evidence of recent infections, these tests should be done on paired samples in the hope of demonstrating a rising titre, although frequently the first sample is taken rather late when the titre is already past the peak. However, a high titre usually indicates recent infection.

In Britain, using the Dye Test, titres in the high hundreds in cats and the low hundreds in dogs are usually considered to be significant. It must be emphasised that the techniques for confirmation of toxoplasmosis infection, with the exception of the latex agglutination test, are complicated and carried out at special laboratories.

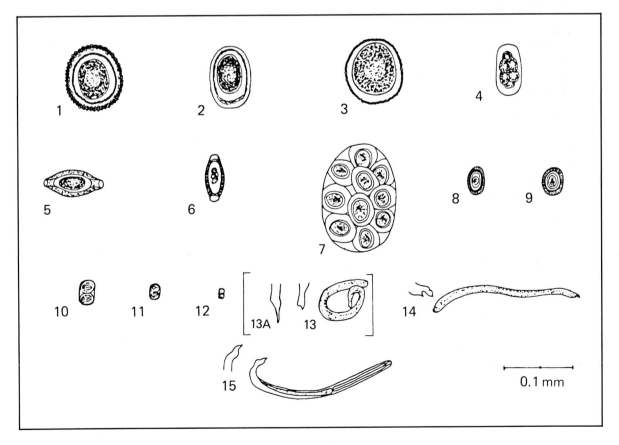

Figure 7.3

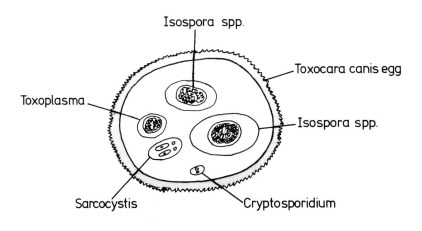

Figure 7.4

INTERPRETATION OF RESULTS

SPECIES DETECTABLE BY ROUTINE FAECES EXAMINATION

Using one or more of the above techniques, eggs or larvae of the following helminths or protozoa of British dogs and cats can be identified (see Figures 7.3 and 7.4).

Intestinal Nematodes

> *Toxocara canis*[1] (dog)
> *Toxascaris leonina*[2]
> *Toxocara cati*[3] (cat)
> *Unicinaria stenocephala*[4]
> *Trichuris vulpis*[5] (dog)
> *Capillaria* spp.[6] (rare)

See illustration of morphological characteristics on page 85.

Intestinal Cestodes (see Figure 7.3)

> *Dipylidium caninum*[7]
> *Taenia* spp.[8]
> *Echinococcus granulosus*[9] (dog)

Intestinal Protozoa

> *Isospora* spp.[10] [11].
> *Toxoplasma gondii*[12] (cat)
> *Cryptosporidia* (Figure 7.4)
> *Sarcocystis* (Figure 7.4)

Respiratory Tract Nematodes

> *Oslerus (Filaroides) osleri*[13] (dog)
> *Filiaroides hirthi*[13A] (exotic sp.)
> *Angiostrongylus vasorum*[14] (dog)
> *Aelurostrongylus abstrusus*[15] (cat)

Morphological characteristics and relative size of the eggs and larvae and, where appropriate, larval tails of the above helminth and protozoal species, are shown in Figures 7.3 and 7.4.

Oocysts found in the faeces of dogs and cats and, indeed, other pets, may be differentiated on morphology, size and stage of development.

Isospora spp. present in fresh faeces of dogs and cats are unsporulated, the larger species being approximately 40 μm x 30 μm and the smaller ones 25 μm x 20 μm. *Sarcocystis* and *Toxoplasma* are 15 x 11 μm and 12 x 10 μm respectively, but are more readily differentiated by the presence of sporocysts or sporulated oocysts in cats infected with *Sarcocystis.*

Cryptosporidium oocysts are very small (4.0 — 4.5 μm) and their detection in faeces requires staining of a faecal smear with Ziehl-Nielsen technique (p.92), the sporozoites appearing as bright red granules.

The relative sizes of these oocysts compared to a *Toxocara* egg are shown in Figure 7.4.

EXOTIC SPECIES

Eggs of the nematodes *Spirocerca lupi*[1] and *Ancylostoma* spp.[2] and the cestode *Diphyllobothrium latum*[3], can also be identified using the above techniques (Figure 7.5) as can the larvae of *Filaroides hirthi*[13A] (Figure 7.3). These are the same size as *O. osleri* but the tail differs.

Where the presence of the lung *(Paragonomus westermani*[4]*)* or liver flukes *(Platynosumum fastosum*[5]*)* are suspected, a flotation solution with a high specific gravity must be used, e.g. zinc sulphate.

Morphological characteristics of eggs from the above exotic species are shown in Figure 7.5.

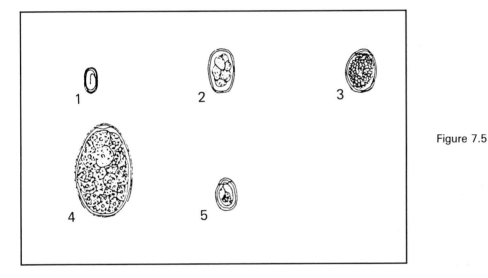

Figure 7.5

INTERPRETATION OF FAECAL ANALYSIS

Several factors must be considered. First, the number of eggs laid by different helminths varies considerably, e.g. high egg counts *Toxocara* or *Toxascaris* eggs are not uncommon, whereas the detection of large numbers of *Oslerus* larvae is rare. Also, the distribution of eggs in faeces is not homogenous and the sample examined may differ from surrounding parts of the faeces collected and great variations occur. Host immunity may depress the egg-laying of the parasites or where immunosuppressive drugs, e.g. steroids are used, the reverse may occur and egg-laying may be enhanced.

Nevertheless, the techniques outlined above do provide a useful adjunct to diagnosis, but must be considered in conjunction with the clinical signs. For a qualitative diagnosis the flotation method using centrifugation probably gives the best result and salt or sugar solutions yield the clearest preparations. Interpretation of the quantitative McMaster method varies for the different species, but counts in excess of 1,000 eggs per gram of nematodes and trematode eggs usually indicate a heavy infection. Counts of protozoal cysts are less meaningful, and it is impossible to quantify cestode infections due to the periodic shedding of segments. It is important to realise that the results of faecal analysis are considered in conjunction with clinical symptoms and the results of other laboratory tests. It is too easy to make a precipitous diagnosis simply in the presence of eggs or larvae in the faeces. As with helminths, the detection of protozoal stages in faeces or blood should not constitute a diagnosis on its own and the findings have to be evaluated in conjunction with clinical signs and other laboratory tests.

OTHER INFORMATION

OTHER PETS

Intestinal helminths and protozoa occur in a wide range of children's pets, and details of these may be found in the B.S.A.V.A. Manual of Exotic Pets. Species which are readily diagnosed by the presence of eggs, oocysts or cysts in the faeces, are as follows:

Rabbits:	*Passalurus ambiguus*	(Oxyuroid-type egg).
	Coccidia oocysts	
Hamsters:	Coccidia oocysts	
	Flagellates & Ciliates	*(Trichomonadas; Hexamita; Giardia; Balantidium).*
Rats & Mice:	*Syphacia obvelata*	
	Aspiculutus tetraptera	
	Coccidia oocysts	
	Hymenolepis nana	*(Taenia*-like eggs).
	Giardia and *Hexamita*	
Tortoises:	Many species of adult and larval nematodes	
	Many flagellates	

The techniques outlined in the section on dogs and cats will detect eggs of any of the above species, though flagellates and ciliates may not survive particularly well in heavily saturated solutions. Indeed, where *Giardia* or *Hexamita* species are suspected the direct smear technique often proves the most reliable. The addition of 2 or 3 drops of 1% methylene blue to the mixture of faeces and water makes detection of these protozoa easier. The trophozoite stages may be recognised by their pear-like shape and an actively motile swimming movement. The flagellae, when present, are only visible when motility becomes sluggish. Cysts appear as colourless, hyaline round bodies rather like coccidia oocyst species. Differentiation of trophozoites or cysts require specialised staining techniques involving alcohol fixation and haematoxylin based stains; final identification is, therefore, probably best made at a parasitology laboratory.

As in dogs and cats, toxoplasmosis of small pets such as rabbits, may be diagnosed by serological tests. Titres considered to be significant in rabbits and guinea pigs are in the thousands, while in rats and mice titres in the hundreds usually indicate active infection.

CHAPTER 8

BACTERIOLOGY

Dr. G. H. K. Lawson B.V.M.&S., Ph.D., B.Sc., M.R.C.V.S.

INTRODUCTION

The aim of this section is to provide a guide to the practitioner on Bacteriology. It does not pretend to be an authoritative treatise on Bacteriology or even Clinical Bacteriology. Many of the clinical deductions made are based on assumptions, consequently they may not always be true but should be valid in the majority of clinical situations. Equally, the information provided for the recognition of organisms may be adequate for clinical assessment but would not satisfy the criteria required in Microbiology.

It is recommended that if a study of a particular problem is undertaken either the more specialised texts are referred to or preferably advice or the assistance of a Microbiologist sought.

Clinical Bacteriology can provide the clinician with information that will indicate the presence or absence of bacterial infection in abnormal tissue, will detect carrier animals that are clinically normal and finally, can provide information on antibacterials likely to be effective in treatment. It is important always to bear in mind, however, that recovery of bacteria from a clinical condition does not necessarily infer that the organism is the cause of the condition. Failure to recover bacteria does not always rule out infection, laboratories vary in the range of procedures normally undertaken, and not all bacteria can be conveniently recovered in culture while inhibitory substances may prevent the recovery of organisms that can usually be cultivated. Bacteriological information cannot be used without thorough clinical assessment.

SAMPLE COLLECTION

Contamination by commensal bacteria that are normally present on the epithelial surfaces of the body is a constant problem associated with sampling and the interpretation of the results of bacteriological analysis. Specific guidance is given in relation to particular tissues later in this section. Samples for analysis should only be taken into sterile containers using sterile instruments; this is so obvious that it should not require statement. However, it has to be remembered that some fibre-optic instruments are not suitable for heat sterilisation and have to be sterilised by chemical means with the additional attendant danger of microbial inhibition.

Samples taken normally comprise swabs that absorb exudate or pus from a lesion, fluid aspirates from blood, body cavities or joints and other body secretions. Swabs are supplied dry or in a relatively inert transport medium, which helps retain the viability of the more fragile bacteria. Samples should be examined or chilled ($+5^{\circ}C$) as soon as possible after they are obtained; delay in examination results in changes in the populations of bacteria in the sample, which may make deductions from the results invalid. The general principles of clear and accurate labelling of each sample that pertains for samples taken for other disciplines, holds for bacteriological samples.

In general, samples from purulent lesions are best taken as an aspirate or on a heavily loaded swab, the former is to be preferred where anaerobic infection is suspected. Transport media is most appropriate when the object is to detect the presence of a specific, often fragile pathogen. However, microbial changes subsequent to sampling may be more profound than in other types of samples. Specific transport media designed for the isolation of groups of bacteria e.g. Mycoplasma or Chlamydia are almost essential if isolation of these agents is required.

Urine Sampling. There is no ideal method of collection. Catheterisation is the best method of obtaining useful samples regularly; care must be taken to maintain asepsis. Prepubic bladder puncture will be undertaken rarely but might be the method of choice for obtaining urine for culture for leptospira. Owners or kennel staff can often take satisfactory mid stream samples during normal urination. Samples should be taken with a small sterile kidney dish and discarded if obvious contamination takes place.

LABORATORY METHODS

ROUTINE PROCEDURES

The examination of clinical specimens for the presence of bacteria follows a fairly well defined pathway involving a number of steps. On occasion, more sophisticated or alternate approaches may be utilised but the outline indicated below is generally appropriate for a sample from a suspected infection of unknown cause.

1. Smear and examine microscopically for bacteria and fungi.

2. Culture specimens taking into account any information obtained from (1). Samples in which bacteria are not seen must also be cultured.

3. Carry out sensitivity tests if indicated.

4. Incubate culture plates, examine and relate to (1).

5. Read sensitivity test or carry out test on colonies now isolated.

6. Where identity of bacteria uncertain or more detailed examination required, sub-culture bacteria to further media for additional tests.

Microscopy

The microscope is one of the foundations upon which diagnostic bacteriology is built. Whilst there is often a temptation to omit the microscopic examination of specimens this should not be done and every care taken to correlate the observations made on the clinical specimen by microscopy and the results obtained by cultural examination. This provides a useful control on technique and often avoids drawing false conclusions from artefacts.

Bacteria, whether in tissues or culture, retain certain stains and, when observed under the oil immersion lens of the microscope, can be seen readily. The organisms of each species possess a characteristic shape due to the rigid cell wall. Too much should not be made of small variations in the shape or size and if the shapes in Figure 8.1 can be appreciated it will suffice.

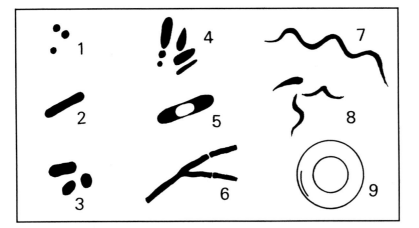

Figure 8.1

1. Cocci
2. Rod or bacilli
3. Cocco-bacilli
4. Pleomorphic cocco-bacilli
5. Bacillus with spore
6. Rods with branching
7. Spirochaete
8. Campylobacters
9. Red blood cell for comparison of size

Normally, bacteria will possess the same shape and size whether growing in culture or when present in tissues. Although small differences may be ignored the bacteria recovered therefore should correlate with those seen in the original tissue.

Preparation and examination of smears

Direct smears from tissues are not always helpful.

Where the tissue is normally sterile or carries a small bacterial population, useful information can be obtained. Where there is a commensal population, pathogens are only likely to be recognised if they differ morphologically from the commensals, stain differently or are sufficiently predominant for their presence to be noticed.

1. **Swabs**
   Make smears from swabs taken from pathological conditions by firmly rolling the swab over the surface of a sterile slide. Hold slide carefully to avoid touching fingers with swab. Where the swab has become dried-out, moisten it in nutrient broth or sterile saline before making smears. Where the cultural procedure for swabs taken from a particular condition or source are standardised, it is probably better to inoculate plates first, thus reducing the possibility of introducing contaminations onto the culture media.

2. **Fluids**
   Transfer 1—2 drops to a slide using bacteriological loop or Pasteur pipette. Spread, allow to air dry. Fluids containing fibrinogen e.g. synovial fluid, are best taken aseptically into heparin, otherwise the bacteria and cells are trapped in the clot that forms subsequently. If anti-coagulant has not been used, smears and cultures should be prepared soon after collection.

3. **Faeces**
   Examine for abnormal constituents. If flakes of tissue or mucus are present remove with a bacteriological loop, emulsify in a little saline on a slide, spread out and air dry.

4. **Biopsy specimens**
   These should be taken aseptically and placed in a sterile container and handled thereafter with sterile instruments. Representative portions are fixed for histology. Cut surfaces should be smeared on a sterile slide and plates inoculated by rubbing the cut surface over the surface of the media. The fungal elements in some mycotic infections are not demonstrated easily, necessitating the digestion of surrounding cells with alkali. A small 1mm block of tissue from the centre of the lesion is crushed between two slides and 2 or 3 drops of 20% KOH added before covering the preparation with a coverslip. The preparation is kept warm and examined at intervals. In some cases it may take many hours before fungal hyphae can be seen. This procedure is important as many of the agents which cause these lesions are prominent in the environment, their appearance, therefore, in culture is not good evidence as to their origin unless either a digest or histology gives evidence of their presence in the tissues.

5. **Tissues at necropsy**
   These are taken similarly to (1) above only it is now possible to fully sterilse the surface of the tissue before sampling — by searing the surface with a hot spatula. Many lesions are quite small and the bacteria may be confined to the lesion and not distributed throughout the tissue. Care taken in selecting lesions is always repaid. Where lesions are progressive the periphery, at the edge of cell reaction, generally gives a better indication of the offending organisms. If in doubt, sample at more than one point and compare results. Portions of tissue are removed with a sterilised bacteriological loop, Pasteur pipette or removed aseptically as in (4).

THE STAINING OF BACTERIA

Slides
It is important that the slide is absolutely clean. Polish with a clean cloth and then heat until too hot to touch.

Staining
The practice laboratory can function adequately with the small number of dyes required to carry out Gram's stain, Ziehl-Neelsen's acid fast stain and any one of the Romanofsky stains used in haematology.

Smears are allowed to dry in air alone or speeded up by mild heat. When dry, fixation for all smears (except those to be stained Romanofsky) is carried out by heat. Pass the dry slide through the bunsen flame a number of times until hot to the touch, allow to cool before staining.

Slides are normally stained suspended on a rack made of two glass rods, over a sink or basin. Water must be available either from a tap or in a wash bottle beside the staining area. Stains are best kept in small dropping bottles.

Stain all smears by Gram's method as a routine. Where clinical symptoms suggest a Mycobacterial infection or where the Gram stain demonstrates inflammatory cells but no obvious bacteria, stain another smear for acid fast organisms. Some bacteria, particularly Gram negative anaerobes, may be best seen by staining with Romanofsky stains. These stains often demonstrate occasional organisms which would be missed amongst inflammatory cells when stained by Gram's. The Brucella differential stain in small animal practice is almost only used in the diagnosis of psittacosis or chlamydial infections.

Where the morphological features of organisms in culture are to be determined, a small amount of a colony is removed and emulsified in sterile saline or distilled water. Such smears should only just be opaque and several such preparations can be made separately on one slide. Slides and smears are identified by marking with a diamond marker.

Gram stain
1. Solutions
    a. Crystal Violet.
    b. Gram's Iodine.
    c. Acetone or Methylated spirits (industrial methyl-alcohol).
    d. Dilute carbol fuchsin (ZN carbol fuchsin diluted 1/10 with distilled water) or Safranine 0.5% in distilled water.

2. Procedure
    a. Flood the slide with crystal violet solution, leave on for 30—60 seconds. (Time not critical).
    b. Wash, drain slide and immediately flood with Gram's iodine, leave for 30—60 seconds.
    c. Wash, drain. Turn on tap water. Flood slide with acetone and immediately wash with water. This is the critical step and acetone is a harsh decolouriser; it does however produce more clear cut results than other decolourisers. With some bacteria (Bacillus and Clostridia) it may be too severe and methylated spirits will give better results. Using methylated spirits, slides are decolourised until the colour ceases to come out of the smear, normally about 30 seconds. The contrast obtained with methylated spirits is less clear than with acetone.
    d. Counterstain with dilute carbol fuchsin or safranine 30—60 seconds. Where dilute carbol fuchsin is being used prolonged staining may cause Gram negative organisms to be mistakenly considered as Gram positive.
    e. Wash, shake off excess water and air dry. Gram's stain colours certain organisms purple-blue and these are called Gram positive; bacteria which are decolourised by acetone and stain red to orange with the counterstain, are called Gram negative. This staining reaction is an important feature in identifying bacteria, but some organisms belonging to Gram positive species sometimes may not stain correctly. With some species only young cultures stain correctly, older cultures appearing as a mixture of Gram positive and negative forms. Similar problems are also encountered in tissue smears where damage to the bacterial cell wall has taken place.

Ziehl-Neelsen acid fast stain
1. Solutions
    a. Carbol Fuchsin.
    b. Acid Alcohol (concentrated hydrochloric acid 3.0ml; ethyl alcohol 97.0ml).
    c. Methylene blue 0.5%.

2. Procedure
    a. Flood smear with Carbol Fuchsin. Heat gently with ignited cotton wool swab previously moistened with methylated spirits. Allow slide to steam, do **not** boil. Leave stain on for 5 minutes and repeat heating.

b.   Rinse off excess stain and flood with acid alcohol. Genuine acid fast bacteria resist decolourisation for more than 5 minutes. Organisms appearing acid fast in tissues and not in culture may be more readily decolourised. During the decolourisation process the acid alcohol is refreshed on two occasions.

c.   Rinse with water and counterstain with methylene blue for 30 seconds. Wash, shake off excess water and dry. Acid fast bacteria appear bright red on a blue background, methylene blue stains tissue cells and other bacteria.

Modified Ziehl-Neelsen stain

The main application of this stain in small animal practice is in the diagnosis of psittacosis in cage birds.

The cut surface of the excised spleen is lightly dabbed on to a slide. Remove excess blood first by blotting before making impression smears. (Dispose of the contaminated blotting paper carefully in disinfectant). Air dry and fix in the normal way, cool slide before staining.

1.   Solutions
   a.   Dilute Carbol Fuchsin.
   b.   0.5% Acetic Acid.
   c.   Methylene Blue 0.5%.

2.   Procedure
   a.   Flood slide with dilute Carbol Fuchsin for 10 minutes.
   b.   Wash with water and decolourise with 0.5% acetic acid for 20—30 seconds. This is the critical stage and, when properly stained, the normal cells in the finished stained smear should just demonstrate an occasional pink blush.
   c.   Counterstain lightly with methylene blue for 20 seconds. When positive for psittacosis, tissue cells will be observed containing clusters of red bodies in which the individual bodies are so small as to be at the limit of resolution of light microscopes.

MEDIA

Bacteria are grown on solid media where each bacterium is capable of multiplying to form a visible colony on the surface. These bacterial colonies tend to have a typical appearance depending on the species; most are roughly circular with a more or less raised centre. Culturing bacteria allows more precise identification and allows sensitivity tests to antibacterial substances to be carried out on clinical isolates.

Media can be purchased as ready poured plates (see appendix) or prepared in the practice laboratory.

Types of Media

A fluid media which includes all the nutrients required to grow bacteria are included, is called a broth. The second type of media consists of a nutrient solution made solid by the addition of agar. This substance is inert as far as micro-organisms are concerned, melts at 95°C and solidifies to a gel at 42°C. The latter property allows heat sensitive nutrients to be added to the media without damage after the media has been melted. Solid media is most commonly poured in flat dishes with lids, called plates, and are made of glass or plastic. Certain media are selective i.e. have substances included to inhibit the growth of commensal organisms which tend to overgrow pathogens in culture.

Some Media and their Uses

Media	Use
Plates: Blood Agar	Standard solid media, will support growth of most pathogens.
McConkey Agar	Selective media for enteric pathogens.
Deoxycholate Citrate Agar	Selective media for growing Salmonellae.
Sabourauds' Chloramphenicol Agar	Media suitable for most ringworms or other fungal infections.

Some Media and their Uses *(continued)*

Media	Use
Broths: Nutrient Broth	Standard broth for growing bacteria in fluid culture.
Glucose Broth	Enriched broth for growing Streptococci.
Selenite F Broth	Selective broth for growing Salmonellae.

Whilst the purpose of both fluid and solid media is to support the growth of micro-organisms, solid agar media has one major advantage in that it allows some assessment of the relative numbers of different kinds of bacteria present in the sample to be made. This is not possible with liquid broths and the predominant organisms after 24 hours' incubation in broth need not be the same as that which was most numerous in the lesion. Additionally, broth culture gives little indication of the numbers of organisms present in the original tissue. For this reason, primary broth cultures are generally reserved for those tissues in which the numbers of the pathogen are small and contaminants are absent. The exception is the use of selective broth media for the recovery of pathogens present in small numbers in the original sample.

Sterilisation

All media must be sterilised before inoculation. This is commonly achieved by heat treatment, filtration or deriving the fluid aseptically from an animal source. Most basal media are available commercially and this is the source of choice; no small laboratory can hope to adequately test the performance of media. Media are supplied generally as a powder or in tablet form. These are rehydrated according to the manufacturer's instructions, boiled to dissolve and then sterilised by autoclaving. The essential equipment consists of a small autoclave, similar to those used for surgical dressings, and glassware (conical flasks and medical flats). Agar media can often be pre-prepared without disadvantage, in this the basal media is sterilised in screw capped glass containers and stored until required. Immediately before use the media is melted in a boiling water bath, cooled to 50°C and any necessary ingredients included before pouring. Most perishable media ingredients, serum or blood, can also be purchased from manufacturers. In many cases these can be stored frozen for long periods although if blood is frozen it becomes useless for the detection of bacterial haemolysis.

Storage

A problem of small laboratories with irregular demands is how best to store media. Bottled fluid media will keep almost indefinitely at +5°C, plates of solid agar media tend to dry out, even if kept at +5°C, and become unsatisfactory with time (3—6 weeks). This period can be prolonged by chilling the plates to +5°C then packing in polythene bags and storing the packed plates at +5°C.

CULTURE TECHNIQUES

There will always be some bacteria and fungi present in the laboratory environment. Specific steps are needed to ensure that these are not introduced accidentally into the media used. The following important instruments and techniques are used in transferring micro-organisms in the laboratory.

Instruments

Bacteriological loop. This is used for plating out cultures or pathological specimens and in transferring fluid cultures to plates and vice versa. Sterilisation is by heating the wire loop to red heat. Although only the loop portion is used for inoculation, the complete sterilisation of the whole wire at the start of inoculation procedures avoids accidentally introducing organisms into the neck of containers.

Capillary pipettes

The capillary end is sterilised by heat, the pipette allowed to cool and a rubber teat attached to the other end. These pipettes are very useful for transferring larger volumes of fluid aseptically and in other laboratory manipulations.

Inoculation

Prior to inoculation the surface of the plates should be checked for contaminants and discarded if any are present.

When preparing primary plates from pathological material the inoculum should be spread over a quarter of the plate (A, Figure 8.2.i). The loop is then sterilised by flaming and the inoculum spread out further by drawing the loop over the surface of the plate in the direction of the arrow. (ii) Resterilise the loop and continue to (iii) and (iv). This is probably the single most important step in diagnostic bacteriology. The important object is to separate the individual bacteria on the plate so that after incubation they grow into well separated individual colonies — not just an indeterminate mass.

Inoculation of broths with bacteria (as opposed to pathological material) is carried out by picking up a portion of the colony by wire or loop. The inoculum is emulsified in the broth just above the fluid line. Ensure inoculation is complete by detecting the slight opacity due to bacteria on the wall of the container. Selective media should be inoculated with considerably more material than the equivalent non-selective media.

Incubator and incubation

Most pathogenic bacteria and fungi will grow over a range of temperatures. The rate of growth and therefore, colony size is an important feature in their recognition. The normal incubator temperature is 37°C (thermostatically controlled) which is adequate for most purposes although specific organisms may be more easily isolated at different temperatures.

For most purposes media should be incubated for 5 days at 37°C (34—40°C) before discarding as negative. This procedure can be modified with experience. Plates are incubated with the media on top and the lid on the bottom of the incubator or shelf.

i 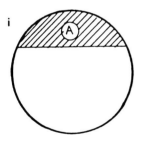   ii 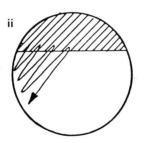   iii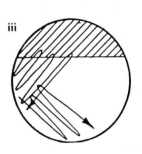

iv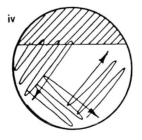

Figure 8.2

Table 8.1
Some commonly isolated bacteria and their simple features

Colony Diameter	Colony Colour, Shape	Haemolysis on Blood Agar	Bacterial Shape	Growth on MacConkey Agar 1 †	Catalase	Possible Identity
2 mm or more at 18h	White or cream	+ or −	G + cocci	Icing sugar like, may appear as red (LF) pink or yellow (NLF)	+	*Staphylococcus aureus* Coagulase + or *Staphylococcus epidermidis* Coagulase−
2mm approx. at 18h	White	−	G + cocci or oval or short bacilli	Smaller than BA Flat colonies, LF +ve	−	Intestinal cocci, the enterococci
2 mm or more at 18h	Grey or Grey/White	+ or −	G−bacilli	LF +ve, colonies almost same size as BA		Coliforms; if from genital, urinary or intestinal tract, probably *Escherichia coli*
2 mm approx at 18h	Grey	−	G−bacilli	NLF, colonies almost same size as BA		Possibly *Salmonella* — see tests
2 mm or more at 18h	Grey, with or without green pigment dif- fusing into the media, smell	−	G−bacilli	NLF, often distinctive brownish colony pigment and irregular edge		*Psuedomonas aeruginosa*
2 mm or more at 18h	Grey, white often irregular	+ or −	G+bacilli	Variable		*Bacillus,* cultures should show spores if incubation prolonged
Spreading in waves across plate	Grey	−	G−bacilli	NLF, 2 mm, edge of colony may tend to spread		*Proteus*
2 mm approx.	Grey	−	G−bacilli small and often cocco- bacillary	Slight or absent		*Pasteurella* or Pasteurella-like*
0.5 - 2 mm	Translucent to white		G+cocci	Absent. Some urinary strains grow	−	*Streptococci.* Generally serological group G, C or L if significant
0.5 - 2 mm	Grey	−	G−coccobacilli	Absent		Isolated from genito-urinary *Haemophilus.* Fails to grow on media without added blood
Less than 0.5 mm at 18h growing to 2 mm at 48h	Grey/White	−	G−bacilli	Size as for BA NLF		Possibly *Bordetella bronchiseptica* if isolated from respiratory tract
Less than 0.5 mm at 18h growing to 2 mm at 48h	Grey/White	−	G−small bacilli	Size as for BA NLF		From intestinal tract, possibly *Yersinia pseudotuberculosis*
Colonies minute at 18h increasing to 1-2 mm at 48h	White, often rough, or irregular	−	G+small bacilli Often bizarre, pleomorphic and coccal forms	Absent		*Corynebacteria,* often loosely called diphtheroids
Colonies not visible at 18h becoming visible after 48h	White, often rough or irregular	−	G+delicate bacilli Acid fast G+bacilli branching forms			*Mycobacteria* *Nocardia*

† NLF: *Non-lactose fermenting pale or yellow colonies;* LF: *Lactose fermenting pink or red.*
* *If from pathological material, it is likely to be Pasteurella or Pasteurella-like.*
  Where recovery from other source, identification uncertain and needs further tests.

IDENTIFICATION OF BACTERIA

1. Record all steps taken in the examination of a specimen, e.g. what is seen in smear, the appearance of colonies that grow and details of tests carried out. Number all plates on the base, identifying if primary plates or sub-cultures.

2. Examine colonies growing on primary plates (see Table 8.1).

3. Assess which bacterial colonies may be involved in the clinical condition. This is generally done either on numerical predominance or the presence of a specific pathogen. Only a limited number of bacterial species can be identified by the appearance of the colonies. Organisms are commonly identified by a combination of colony appearance, cell morphology, physiological and biochemical characters and surface antigens. Subculture single colonies to ensure pure growth.

4. Confirm microscopic appearance of bacteria if necessary and carry out further specific identification procedures.

5. In many cases the identification of an organism is not relevant to the management of the case. For instance, a well taken urinary sample which shows Gram-negative bacilli and inflammatory cells and yields a Gram-negative bacillus on culture may need no further assessment than the sensitivity of the bacteria to antimicrobials. However, even here on the occasion of failure to respond to treatment, identification may help separate reinfection of the bladder from failure of therapy. In many instances correct identification is the only guide that differentiates commensals from pathogens. Once the basic cultural and morphologic properties of an organism have been established, reliance is often placed on the ability of the organism to utilise substrates, different species of bacteria having different activities. Composite media that allow identification are available commercially. Using such kits, bacteria can be characterised at a fraction of the cost of the preparation of individual media but not without moderate expense.

    A range of kits are required to identify the range of bacterial species likely to be encountered; the kits have a reasonable shelf life. Manufacturers supply detailed instructions for the use of the kits, the identification of bacteria based on their results, and some will readily provide assistance in case of difficulty (see page 145). Identification has generally proved satisfactory with human strains, but not all animal pathogens may be identified accurately.

Identification tests

The following tests may prove useful on occasion for the identification of some of the more commonly occurring pathogens of the dog or cat. They relate to those characters mentioned in Table 8.1.

Catalase Test Place a small portion of growth on slide, add one drop 3% Hydrogen Peroxide. Positive reaction if bubbles result. (Weak catalase producers may show false negative).

DNA'se Test Pathogenic Staphylococci produce large amounts of DNA'se. *Staphylococcus intermedius*, the common pathogen of the dog and cat, in addition to DNA'se production grow as white colonies and are variable in demonstrating clumping factor. *Staphylococcus aureus* is yellow pigmented, always produces clumping factor and is coagulase positive. Staphylococcal strains are grown overnight on DNA agar at 37°C, residual DNA is precipitated by N-HCl allowing DNA'se production to be visualised as a clear zone surrounding the colonies.

Clumping Factor (Slide coagulase test). Add rabbit plasma on a straight wire to a dense suspension of bacteria in water on a slide. A positive reaction is indicated by clumping after 5 seconds.

Coagulase Test. Confirmatory — Tube Test — To 0.5ml of 1/10 dilution of rabbit plasma in saline add 0.1 ml of an 18—24 hour broth culture of the organism. Incubate at 37°C and examine at 1, 3, and 6 hours and after overnight incubation at room temperature. A definite clot is formed by coagulase positive organisms. Positive and negative control cultures are essential as plasma is unstable. Dried rabbit plasma is available commercially, keep reconstituted plasma at +5°C (not frozen).

Precipitin tests (Streptococci). Acid Extraction — Inoculate glucose broth with organism under investigation, incubate overnight at 37°C.

Centrifuge and discard supernatant into disinfectant, add 0.5 ml N/20 HCl 1/200 dilution of concentrated HCl) and place in a water bath for 10 minutes. Cool and add 2 drops phenol red indicator (0.02%). Add just sufficient N-NaOH to turn the indicator red, centrifuge and use the supernatant as antigen. Draw up streptococcal antiserum into a tapered capillary tube by placing the tip of the capillary tube in the serum. (Figure 8.3). Place tube upright in plasticine block and carefully add prepared antigen with a very finely drawn out pipette. It is important that the antigen forms a distinct layer on top of the serum. A fine white ring of precipitate forms at interface in a positive reaction within 15 minutes. Observe by viewing the capillary against a dark background with overhead lighting.

The precipitin test requires technical dexterity and alternative tests employing serum sensitised latex particles or Staphylococcal cells in a slide agglutination procedure may be more satisfactory but expensive alternatives. (See Appendix, page 145).

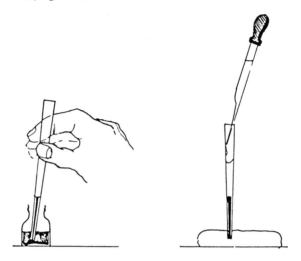

Figure 8.3

Identification of Salmonellae. The culture procedure described will isolate from faeces many but not all of the clinically significant salmonellae. Organisms growing to well developed colonies within 18 hours and failing to ferment lactose (clear or yellow on McConkey or deoxycholate citrate agar) which are Gram-negative bacilli may be salmonellae.

Sub-culture suspect colonies to McConkey agar for serological testing. A portion of the resultant growth is removed and emulsified in saline on a slide. The suspension should not be so dense as to restrict the flow when the slide is tilted; nor should it be too light, otherwise positive reactions may be missed. A drop of Polyvalent Salmonella 'O' is added and the slide tilted back and forward observing the drop with a dark background and indirect overhead light. A positive reaction (Figure 8.4) is indicated by clumping. A positive reaction indicates either:

(a) The organism is a Salmonella

(b) It is a related organism

(c) The organism is unstable and will clump even in the absence of serum.

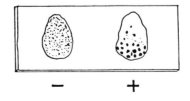

Figure 8.4

To confirm as a Salmonella, test again in slide agglutination tests with specific 'O' antisera. Normally Group B (0 4), Group C (0, 6 and 7) and Group D (0 9) antisera will suffice. A positive reaction with one of these indicates a Salmonella and it should be sent to a suitable laboratory for final identification; a positive reaction to more than one serum indicates that the organism is unstable [see (c)]. A negative reaction indicates that the organism is probably not a Salmonella and in these cases the original Polyvalent reaction was probably weak. Alternatively, it may be a Salmonella which does not belong to Groups B, C, and D and in this case confirmation can be obtained by the use of multi-media kits for biochemical testing, a number of which are available commercially (Appendix). Where positive confirmation of identity has been made on an early isolate by a reference laboratory, a procedure such as the above may usefully be used to monitor infection or excretion without necessitating recourse to full identification on each occasion.

Procedure for Examination of Faeces

1. Obtain rectal faeces. Examine for abnormal contents, blood, mucus, etc.
2. Smear and stain Gram's.
3. Inoculate blood agar, McConkey agar and Deoxycholate citrate agar (DCA) and Campylobacter selective media (incubated microaerobially).
4. Inoculate 10 ml Selenite F broth with ½ to 1 gram faeces.
5. After 18—24 hours incubation take 3 or 4 loopfuls from the Selenite F broth and inoculate a new DCA plate.
   Examine primary DCA plate and the subculture from Selenite F broth for non-lactose fermenting colonies.
6. After 48 hours, examine Campylobacter medium for mucoid colonies with cells of Campylobacter morphology.

Sensitivity tests (Disc Test)

Such procedures attempt to predict the outcome of treatment of an infection involving bacteria with antimicrobial drugs. Tests are carried out by inoculating the surface of a plate with the pathogen and then applying discs, impregnated with the antibacterial compound, onto the surface of the plate. Failure of the organism to grow round the disc indicates sensitivity to the drug concerned. A number of factors influence the size of the zone of inhibition, the media and the number of bacteria inoculated being the most important. Both should be standardised. The numbers of bacteria inoculated should be adjusted to give a growth which is not quite confluent after overnight incubation (Fig. 5). Too many bacteria inoculated will result in an inaccurate test which generally causes effective drugs to be rejected as ineffective.

The zone size is unrelated to the efficacy of antibacterials. Equally, a zone of inhibition does not mean that the organism will respond clinically. Ideally, compare the zone size of a clinically sensitive strain with the organism under test.

In the practice situation, interpret the test by comparing the zone normally produced by known sensitive organisms to that of the organism under test. Any significant reduction (6mm or more in diameter) is generally taken to indicate potential resistance.

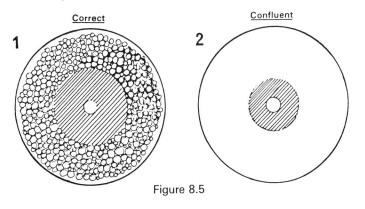

Figure 8.5

1. Direct Sensitivity Tests on Pathological Material

Only applicable where the tissue does **not** have a large resident bacterial population i.e. tissues normally sterile or with low bacterial population.

(a) Examine Gram stained smear. If only one or two bacteria seen, do not carry out test.

(b) Swab smear sample evenly over the culture plate (Figure 8.6). Place a group of sensitivity discs centrally in the plate with sterile forceps.

(c) Incubate overnight at 37°C and read results as sensitive, resistant and intermediate. If growth is too heavy or light, repeat on pure cultures.

(d) Urine samples — inoculate from the 1/100 urine dilution (see Urinary Tract).

(e) If more than one organism is present the sensitivity test of one organism may be influenced by the other. Sensitivity tests may reveal organisms masked by others on the direct blood plate.

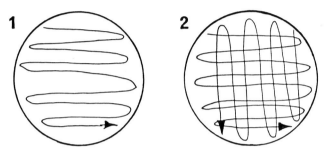

Figure 8.6

2. Sensitivity Test on Organisms in Culture

(a) There should be evidence that the organism is behaving as a pathogen before proceeding.

(b) Pick off 5 representative colonies with a straight wire, emulsify in 1ml sterile saline. With a swab and using the saline suspension, inoculate as in (1).

(c) If the above gives too heavy an inoculum, use a well grown broth culture diluted 1/1000 and proceed as before.

3. General Notes

(a) The use of special sensitivity test agar avoids substances in the media antagonising antibacterials in these tests.

(b) Manufacturers supply discs in different combinations attached together.

(c) It is customary to test drugs active in urinary tract infections using higher level discs, otherwise clinical activity against some bacteria may be missed.

(d) Penicillinase-producing staphylococci fail to grow round penicillin discs but may be detected by the appearance of full sized colonies at the edge of inhibition. Such strains are normally considered resistant.

Sensitivity Tests (Alternative Methods).

Sensitivity to antimicrobials can also be assessed by directly evaluating the minimum inhibitory concentration of the drug (M.I.C.). This involves incorporating the drugs in the media at a variety of concentrations in separate plates.

Plates are then seeded with the organisms to be tested and incubated in the normal manner. Whilst such tests give a more accurate assessment of the M.I.C. it is still difficult to choose the concentration of drug that indicates the organism to be clinically resistant. Manufactured procedures involving this principal are available; all are designed for human use.

Aerobic or Microaerobic Culture

A high percentage of clinical samples contain anaerobic as well as aerobic bacteria. Systems are available that provide anaerobic or microaerobic conditions without a supply of hydrogen or use of a vacuum pump and some replace the standard anaerobic jar with plastic envelopes. These advances make anaerobic and microaerobic culture possible in a practice laboratory.

EXAMINATION OF CLINICAL SAMPLES AND INTERPRETATION OF RESULTS

Skin

1. Select a recently developed or the periphery of an extending, established lesion. Where these are vesicular or pustular choose an unruptured lesion if possible.

2. Clip excess hair from the lesion site.

3. Where the lesion is closed, clean with alcoholic solution and allow to dry. This may not be possible or desirable with open lesions; disinfectant solutions should not be used as contamination of the sample may preclude the recovery of the organisms responsible.

4. Where the lesion is exudative, sample with a sterile swab; where proliferative, scrape periphery of lesion with a scalpel held at right angles to the tissue. Ensure that any damaged or broken hairs are included. Inoculate plates appropriately then transfer the remainder of the samples to two clean slides, smear one and allow to dry for staining Gram. To the second slide add two drops of 10% KOH and apply a coverslip. Examine with the x 10 or x 20 objective for either fungal hyphae or the presence of spores, concentrating on that proportion of the hair that normally lies within the hair follicles. An accurate diagnosis can be made only if the spores are **reasonably numerous**. Air bubbles, oil or drops of emulsion may all mimic spores.

The criteria most useful for differentiating these physical forms from spores, is the variability in size of the former. In freshly taken and examined samples, fungal hyphae if observed are likely to be significant. If a diagnosis cannot be made by direct microscopy, the sample must be cultured. The most likely causes of inconclusive microscopy are the visualisation of small numbers of possible spores or of the failure to demonstrate dermatophytes in a lesion that clinically resembles ringworm. Scrapings should be taken from the periphery of the lesion taking care to include plucked hair and these submitted for culture. Where enough possible cases are seen to justify culture diagnosis within the practice this can be undertaken without difficulty and the techniques are well described.

Cultures of superficial cutaneous lesions can help in establishing if there is significant bacterial infection of the lesion. Recovery of bacteria in significant numbers from skin lesions does not imply that these organisms initiated the change; it only indicates that infection is one facet of the dermatitis which needs attention and appropriate treatment.

Staphylococcus intermedius often predominates in superficial infections and this species is one in which acquired resistance is commonplace. Sensitivity testing is therefore important in the treatment of refractory conditions.

Establishing the presence or absence of infection is straightforward when samples from normally dry and clean skin are examined. This is not so when examining, say, feet or perineal lesions and in these places it may be most difficult to assess whether the bacteria recovered are genuinely playing a part in the course of the disease. Where a number of sites are involved in lesions of this type, sample several and compare results.

Vaccines. Autogenous vaccines may be used to treat chronic recurrent pyoderma. Make a primary culture as soon after sampling as possible. Submit subcultures made from the predominant colonies, together with the primary plates, to the preparing laboratory.

Uncommon Infections. Ulcerative or nodular skin lesions may occur due to Mycobacteria in the dog, cat, primates or zoo animals. Varying numbers of acid fast bacteria may be seen in smears made from the lesions. These organisms may be *M. tuberculosis, M. bovis, M. lepraemurium,* other pathogenic mycobacteria or merely commensals.

Ears

Inflammation of the ears of the cat and rabbit are predominantly of parasitic origin. In the dog, it is common to find only microbial agents in association with otitis externa. The part played by these organisms in the initiation of the lesion is uncertain but a resolution is likely to be delayed in the presence of large numbers of bacteria and fungi.

Pityrosporum appears most commonly in the external ear. They are Gram positive pear-shaped bodies $5-10\mu$ in diameter (considerably larger than the bacteria). Unlike other yeasts, most strains of *Pityrosporum* do not grow well on routine bacteriological or fungal media. *Staphylococci, Enterococci, Streptococci, Diphtheroids, Proteus* and *Pseudomonas* are commonly found in otitis externa, the last two being frequently encountered in refractory cases.

Cellulitis and Myositis

Procurement of samples and disinfection methods are similar to those used for skin. Common bacteria associated with such conditions are *Staphylococcus intermedius*, Streptococci, Bacteriodes (gram negative non-sporing anaerobic bacteria) and uncommonly *Actinomyces* sp. Organisms may be plentiful in acute cellulitis but assessing their significance in chronic persistent cellulitis cases with multiple discharging sinuses, is difficult. In the latter, causal organisms may be few in number and it is not simple to differentiate between a persistent cellulitis due to infection and a foreign body cellulitis in which bacteria are multiplying in the exudate. Take all available information into account including the specific identification of the *Staphylococcus* as *intermedius* or *aureus* and the pattern of antibiotic resistance from prior treatment. Myositis is an occasional sequelae to internal fixation of the long bones, commonly involved are *Clostridium welchi and Staphylococcus* sp. The former will be seen as short robust Gram positive bacilli without spores in smears from the wound exudate. They will not grow in aerobic cultures.

Corynebacterium equi may occur occasionally as a cause of persistent cellulitis, the large mucoid colonies are distinct from the other diphtheroids of the cat or dog.

The Eye

Conjunctivitis. Conjunctivitis may be associated with bacteria, frequently Staphylococci or diphtheroids. An infectious feline conjunctivitis is caused by *Chlamydia psittaci;* conjunctival smears, stained Giemsa, in the acute phase, show intracytoplasmic inclusions within conjunctival epithelial cells. Conventional microscopy is unlikely to provide convincing results in chronic or relapsing cases, commercially available reagents are available for immunofluorescent diagnosis which is much more sensitive. Culture is possible but many laboratories do not normally undertake chlamydial isolation.

Respiratory Tract

Rhinitis. Nasal discharge, often in association with canine distemper. Many persistent canine rhinitis cases, without signs of distemper, yield heavy bacterial growths generally *Staphylococcus intermedius* or *aureus* or a variety of Gram negative species, the significance of these isolates is generally unresolved but Staphylococcal species may be carried at this site without symptoms. Persistent rhinitis in young dogs may be associated with mycotic infection. Sometimes *Aspergillus fumigatus* may be cultured from the nasal discharge; *A. fumigatus* is not often recovered from non-infected nasal cavities of urban dogs, a positive culture therefore is highly suggestive despite ubiquity of the agent. This fungus is unlikely to be cultured unless fungal selective media is employed that will suppress bacterial growth. In established cases it may be difficult to recover the fungus from nasal swabs, although the infection can be shown to persist in turbinates or sinuses. Confirm doubtful cases by serology, submit clotted blood samples for precipitin tests to reference laboratories.

Pharyngitis. Invariable plating of pharygeal swabs yields a heavy growth of a number of different species of bacteria each of which is of unknown significance or pathogenicity. Sensitivity testing is likely to be of little value.

Bronchitis. In the dog, most cases are probably primarily a demonstration of canine distemper or other viral infection in which *Bordetella bronchiseptica* is sometimes implicated in the clinical symptoms observed.

B. bronchiseptica may itself induce a bronchitis and be responsible for some outbreaks of 'kennel cough'. During the bonchitic phase, it can be recovered from the nose by plating on conventional blood and McConkey agar.

Recovery of *B. bronchiseptica* does not exclude distemper but equally may be the agent primarily responsible for the symptoms.

Pleurisy. The most important, although uncommon, causes of pleurisy in the adult dog are Actinomycosis, Nocardiosis and Tuberculosis with the former conditions also affecting the cat. Sample pleural fluid by vacutainer. Dispose of needles and adaptors used with **great care.** (In both conditions effusion contains red blood cells. Differentiate from traumatic haemothorax), Appropriately stained smears establish presence of inflammatory cells. Proceed to:

Centrifuge a portion of the exudate at 3000 rpm for 15 minutes. Carefully decant the supernatant into disinfectant. Smear the deposit thickly, air dry, stain and examine for acid fast bacteria. Add sterile saline to the deposit in a screw capped container. Shake and examine fluid with bottle horizontal. Search for flecks or granules. If seen remove with Pasteur pipette or loop, smear by crushing with another slide and stain Gram. *Nocardia* and *Actinomyces* are often present in demonstrable numbers only in these microcolony granules and are not present in any numbers in the remainder of the pleural fluid. Some samples contain flecks of fat and fibrin which resemble the bacterial granules to the naked eye. Microscopy is necessary to resolve this difference. Both aerobic filamentous organisms *(Nocardia)* and microaerophilic organisms *(Actinomyces)* are thought to be involved in these lesions, with the latter more common in abscessation and the former in pleurisy. *Actinomyces* are often difficult to recover culturally from clinical material during life. Demonstration of acid-fast bacteria typical of *M. tuberculosis* in smears from exudative pleurisy or pericarditis are grounds for euthanasia. Acid-fast bacteria may be scarce in such tubercular lesions and easily missed on cursory examination.

Sometimes Nocardia or Actinomycotic infections may involve a mixture of bacterial species frequently obligate Gram negative anaerobic rods (Bacteroides or Fusobacterium). Recent penetrating wounds of the oesophagus also may result in multiple species bacterial infection in which anaerobic bacteria predominate. Microscopy and/or anaerobic culture is therefore an essential component of investigation of pleurisy.

Pneumonia. Most pneumonias in the dog and cat have a primary viral aetiology. The problem of diagnosis is that of elucidating which of the agents capable of initiating the disease is involved, rather than that of identifying which other micro-organisms are present. It is difficult to relate the presence or organisms recovered from the oropharynx with what is developing in the diseased lung and, therefore, to justify bacteriological sampling. If sampling is to be carried out, swab the larynx or obtain tracheal exudate in suitable sedated patients. Such samples are considered to be a satisfactory reflection of the bacterial population of the diseased lung.

Occasional cases of genuine persistent *Pseuodomonas aeruginosa* infection occur but this is usually in association with some underlying pulmonary pathology. Repeated recovery of such an organism may, therefore point to a primary lung abnormality which is not necessarily infectious.

Alimentary Tract

Gingivitis and stomatitis in the dog and cat are commonly associated with increased numbers of bacteria which may promote the development and severity of lesions. The gingival crevice has a large bacterial and spirochaetal population in the healthy animal. There is no evidence that any specific organism is involved in initiating lesions, rather they appear to be the multiplication of organisms normally present in the oral cavity. The appearance of spirochaetes in numbers in oral lesions may be purely the multiplication of these bacteria in damaged or devitalised tissue outwith their normal habitat, the dental crevice. The rest of the alimentary canal also contains its resident flora which remains fairly stable in the mature animal and consists mainly of *E. coli, Cl welchi, Streptococci, lactobacilli* and members of the genus *Bacteroides.* All these organisms will therefore be recovered from the faeces if appropriate techniques are employed.

Evidence incriminating certain strains of *E. coli* as the cause of diarrhoea in the dog and cat is not substantial. Research does not indicate that they are a common cause of diarrhoea in mature animals and even those strains that possess pathogenic properties cannot be recognised easily in the practice laboratory as the antigenicity of adhesive antigens is largely unknown. Commercial tests are available for the detection of heat labile toxin but are probably not suitable for canine strains, such tests also do not detect strains that only produce stable toxin. The diagnosis of *E. coli* diarrhoea in the dog is therefore unsatisfactory at the present time.

Organisms of the genus *Salmonella* from the faeces of a pet does not necessarily mean that it is the cause of the symptoms observed; such an isolation may, however, have importance as a potential source of infection for the owner or his household.

Recovery of members of the genus *Campylobacter* falls into a similar category. These bacteria are microaerophilic requiring reduced amounts of oxygen (6%) before satisfactory growth is obtained. Relatively simple apparatus for producing such atmospheres is available as are the antibiotic supplements required to prepare selective media. Different *Campylobacter sp* can be recovered from dogs, only *C. jejuni* is important as a human pathogen.

Most dog faeces whether diarrhoeic or not, do not contain appreciable numbers of spirochaetes, whilst a small proportion of dogs with chronic diarrhoea do. These organisms can be seen most easily on conventionally Gram stained thin smears of faecal suspensions.

Urinary Tract : Nephritis

Leptospirosis. Canine renal leptospirosis is most commonly associated with serotype *canicola* which organism is excreted freely in the urine. These organisms will not stain with conventional bacterial stains and are best visualised in dark field preparations in freshly taken urine samples. If delay is anticipated the urine should be diluted with an equal volume of neutral phosphate buffer saline and chilled. Alternatively, a drop of formalin should be added to 10 mls of urine. Centrifugation (unless sophisticated differential techniques are employed) is undesirable, because if renal damage is clinically evident, there will be so much debris deposited as to make dark field visualisation difficult. Formalised urine samples may not be easy to interpret as the characteristic motility by which leptospira are recognised is destroyed.

Spirochaetes may not be present in the urine in the early stages of illness but are always likely to be present 10 days after the commencement of symptoms. Antibacterial therapy may suppress excretion which may reappear following withdrawal of treatment. In the absence of treatment the numbers of leptospira decrease with time but may persist, generally at a low level for years. Whilst renal localisation with *canicola* is pronounced this is not so with *icterohaemorrhagiae* or other serotypes and these organisms may not be detectable in urine samples.

Where it is desirable to confirm the diagnosis of leptospirosis by culture, which is the only absolutely certain method of identifying the serotype involved, a laboratory with experience of handling and culturing leptospira should be contacted before samples are taken or the death of the animals is anticipated. At all times when handling urine samples or tissues from possible cases of leptospirosis, **great care must be exercised.**

Serological Diagnosis of Leptospirosis

The antigens of the leptospira are complex and individual serotypes vary in the antigens which they share with other serotypes. A serum titre to a particular serotype does not, therefore, necessarily indicate that infection has taken place with that serotype although in the case of *canicola* a positive titre taken in association with appropriate symptoms is good evidence.

Serological titres should be well developed within ten days of the onset of symptoms and reach high levels (1/3000 to 1/30,000) at this time, falling approximately tenfold within a year. Vaccination will interfere with the interpretation of serological results. However, even with multiple immunisation the serum titre will generally have returned to negative levels one year after the last booster dose.

Clotted blood samples (1—2 ml) should be submitted to the laboratory carrying out the test. Where animals for export require certification, the sample should be submitted to the appropriate laboratory of the Ministry of Agriculture, Fisheries and Food.

Dark Field Microscopy. Ideally, the dark field microscope would only be used for this purpose, however, unless frequent use is made of it, this is not likely to be justified. A simple dark field microscope can be produced by inserting a central stop at the bottom of the condenser. This is cheap and adequate for use with x 10 objectives provided that the microscope illumination is adequate. For use with higher objectives a special dark field condenser is required. These can now be interchanged with ordinary light condensers without difficulty and it takes a matter of minutes to set this up. Detailed instructions for setting up these condensers are given in microscopy texts.

Dark field microscopy causes light to be scattered from the surfaces of objects so that the object is seen brightly lit against a black background. Other bacteria are also visualised but its main use is for demonstrating the leptospira which are not readily demonstrated any other way.

Dark Field Examination of Urine. Place a drop of urine on a slide. Gently place coverslip on top. Examine with x 10 or x 20 objective using dark field illumination. Large numbers of leptospira may be detected with x 10 objectives but normally smaller numbers will require a x 20 objective for clear differentiation from other material. It is difficult to differentiate tissue fibrils from leptospira and the characteristic motility or coils of the leptospira must be demonstrated if doubt exists. Urine samples from male dogs often contain sperm with the heads and tails separated, the latter may be confused by the inexperienced with leptospira (Figure 8.7). A proportion of leptospira will be found with button hook ends, this is a useful character when organisms are dead or non-motile.

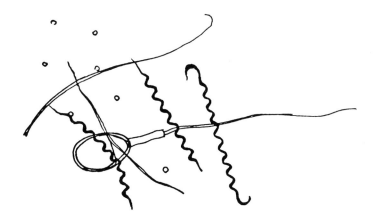

Figure 8.7

Cystitis. Bladder urine in the 'normal' dog or cat is free from bacteria and the appearance of micro-organisms in this fluid must be considered abnormal. The terminal urethra in both male and female contains a significant population of bacteria. The difference between the two sites being mainly maintained by the normal flushing activity of urine. Urine supports the growth of common pathogenic organisms like a bacteriological broth.

As the majority of urine samples obtained will contain some bacteria, the subsequent handling of the specimen is important if a correct interpretation is to be gained. A number of techniques available to evaluate the results of urine culture are based on some assessment of numbers of bacteria in the sample. Most commonly bacteriuria occurs in the canine and the organisms commonly encountered are *E. coli. Proteus* sp., *Staph. intermedius* and B-haemolytic group G Streptococci. When significant, these are present in almost pure culture. The appearance of mixed cultures or organisms not listed may have resulted from the multiplication of contaminating bacteria. Some cultures of urine will yield organisms that grow slowly or irregularly, these may grow better at room temperature than at 37°C and are of no significance.

Bladder infection may or may not relate to the presence of urinary calculi, and occurs more commonly in the bitch. In many cases the cystitis originates from the impedance of the urinary flow by the calculi. However, the frequent association between *Staph. intermedius* and triple phosphate calculi suggest that this organism may play some part in their formation. For this reason monitor clearance of this organism from the bladder following surgical treatment by repeat culturing of samples.

Treatment of Urine. Most samples will contain some bacteria and therefore the subsequent handling of the specimen is important. The practical criteria for handling are listed below.

1. Immediate examination of the specimen.

2. Immediate preparation of smears to be carried out in conjunction with cultural examination later.

3. Use of commercially prepared media which can be inoculated at the time the urine sample is obtained without normal bacteriological tools. An example is the 'Dip Stick' (Urocult Limited).

4. Well taken urine samples should only be held at $+5^{\circ}C$ for 24 hours and not more than 4 hours at room temperature.

Microscopic and Cultural Examination.
1. Make a smear from fresh uncentrifuged urine. Stain Gram, examine for bacteria and cells. Where one or more similar organisms are seen in the majority of high power fields they are likely to be significant.

2. Some quantitive assessments of the bacteria present in urine are useful in interpreting the results. The 'Dip Stick' method achieves this or it may be done by making 1/100 dilution of the urine.

3. Plate out neat urine on blood agar conventionally. This sometimes identifies cases of infected prostatitis that are not demonstrated in the culture of diluted urine. Transfer 1 large loopful of urine to 1 ml of sterile normal saline (1/100 dilution). Mix and plate out one loopful of diluted urine without flaming onto blood agar and one loopful onto McConkey agar.

4. Dip a swab in the 1/100 dilution, spread the moistened swab evenly over a sensitivity test plate. Apply the appropriate antibiotic discs.

5. The appearance of more than 10 colonies on the plate inoculated from diluted urine is likely to indicate a significant infection.

6. McConkey agar is employed to detect infection due to *Proteus,* these bacteria swarm over the surface of conventional agar and it is difficult to estimate their numbers and thus their significance. McConkey agar inhibits this swarming tendency.

Examination of Blood

Many bacterial pathogens that occur in the blood cells of small animals are not normally present in the UK. The sole exception is *Haemobartonella felis* which parasitises the red cells of the blood. (For further information see page 63).

Blood Culture: Blood culture is at its most useful in the diagnosis and therapy of endocarditis in the dog. Blood should be collected using full aseptic technique into a syringe or heparinised vacutainer. Although direct plating may be employed the numbers of bacteria in blood are generally low and enrichment culture is necessary for the detection of many infections. Samples should be about 5—10 ml blood except in some miniature breeds. Streptococci are the most common cause of endocarditis. However, other bacteria including anaerobes may be isolated on occasion from other conditions. Blood culture media should support the growth of both aerobes and anaerobes and some incorporate devices which indicate whether bacterial growth has taken place thus reducing subculturing. Broths should be incubated for a minimum of 3 days and preferably subcultured at the end of the incubation period. There is always a danger of the sample being contaminated by non-significant bacteria, repeat samples help verify the significance of isolates. The recovery of Bacillus sp or DNA'se negative Staphylococci often indicates contamination. Whilst bacteraemia associated with endocarditis can be relatively easily demonstrated, bacteraemia associated with other septic foci is often less easily detected.

ADDITIONAL INFORMATION

TEXTS

Clinical Microbiology and Infectious Diseases of the Dog and Cat.
Edited by C.E. Greene, 1984, Philadelphia, USA, W.B. Saunders.

Manual of Small Animal Infectious Diseases.
Edited by J. E. Barlough, 1988, Longman (Churchill, Livingstone).

Hagan and Bruner's Microbiology and Infectious Diseases of Domestic Animals.
J.T. Timoney, J. H. Gillespie, F. W. Scott and J. E. Barlough, 8th edn. 1988. Cornell University Press.

Medical Microbiology. The Practice of Medical Microbiology.
R. Cruickshank, J.P. Duguid, B.F. Marmion and R.H.A. Swain, 1975. Churchill Livingstone.

A Colour Atlas of Microbiology.
R.J. Olds, 1986. Wolfe Medical Atlas.

Essentials of Veterinary Bacteriology and Mycology.
Carter G.R. 1986. Lea and Febiger

Veterinarians Guide to the Laboratory Diagnosis of Infectious Disease.
Carter G.R. 1986, Medical Publishing Co.

CHAPTER 9

VIROLOGY

H. J. C. Cornwell B.V.M.S., Ph.D., M.R.C.V.S.

INTRODUCTION

THE ROLE OF VIROLOGICAL TESTS

There are three situations in which virology can provide a powerful back-up to the practitioner. **Firstly,** there is the diagnosis or confirmation of diagnosis in an individual animal. This type of investigation is of special relevance when the animal has been vaccinated against the disease now diagnosed. In this situation, exemplified by so-called 'breakdowns' of immunity to canine parvovirus and canine distemper, the owner may have a claim against the vaccine manufacturer who, in turn, will demand laboratory confirmation of the clinical diagnosis before agreeing to a settlement. **Secondly,** there is the epidemiological investigation fundamental to the control or eradication of disease in kennels and catteries; cats persistently infected with feline leukaemia virus must be identified and removed from a cattery if infection is to be eliminated. The infected cat is a major hazzard to other in-contact cats but may be clinically normal, hence the necessity for laboratory tests. **Lastly,** there is the monitoring of the efficacy of vaccination, an ever-expanding field which originated largely from disappointment with the performance of the early canine parvovirus vaccines, coupled with a growing realisation that several other well-known vaccines were less efficient than hitherto believed. All the work and all the argument on canine parvovirus vaccines matters nothing to a dog owner if his fully-vaccinated animal succumbs to distemper, a situation which can be prevented by checking serologically that the dog has indeed responded to the distemper component of the vaccine. Obviously, the converse equally applies.

DEMONSTRATION OF VIRUS

In the first and second of the situations just described, demonstration of the virus clearly has a major role to play. The approach to this is essentially pragmatic, the aim being to utilise that characteristic of the virus which provides the most convenient and readily-detectable 'marker' of its presence. Canine parvovirus, for example, is able to agglutinate pig red blood cells when present in sufficient concentration. The haemagglutination test therefore provides a simple and rapid method for demonstrating the presence of canine parvovirus in faeces samples or gut contents taken at the appropriate stage of the disease process, when high concentrations of virus are present in the lumen of the gut. Unfortunately, however, few canine or feline viruses posess markers that are quite as convenient as that. Coronaviruses and rotaviruses, for example, posess a very specific marker but one which can only be revealed by electronmicroscopy; each of these viruses is constructed to its own very specific architectural plan, readily identifiable with the electron microscope, and because both can be present in very large numbers in the faeces of diarrhoeic animals, this technique often provides a rapid diagnosis. This is fortunate because neither of these viruses is easy to grow in the laboratory. The cost and complexity of an electron microscope does, however, limit the application of this technique to just one or two centres!

VIRUS ISOLATION

For various reasons, virus isolation is often of major importance in the diagnosis of disease. **Firstly,** the ability of a virus to produce a cytopathogenic effect in a cell-culture, as well as the type of cytopathogenic effect produced, is sometimes the only suitable marker available for that virus. **Secondly,** by growing the virus, it becomes possible to obtain sufficient of it for identification; the amount present in the swab or tissue sample is generally quite inadequate for that purpose. **Thirdly,** it may reveal differences in the behaviour of various isolates in the laboratory and hence indicate the emergence of new variants. **Lastly,** since isolates can be stored in the properly-equipped laboratory virtually indefinitely, it caters for retrospective investigation should the diagnosis be questioned at a later date. The cytopathogenic effect can be a dramatic event which leaves no room for doubt. Unfortunately, however, some viruses are non- or only poorly cytopathic while others require special types of cell-culture which are not readily obtainable. In diseases such as canine distemper and feline infectious peritonitis, virus isolation is therefore seldom a practical proposition. At the other extreme, feline calicivirus, canine and feline herpes-viruses, and to a slightly lesser extent, the canine adenoviruses are highly cytopathic so that virus isolation is a straightforward and sensitive procedure that seldom fails unless the virus has been inactivated during transit. However, even with feline calicivirus, several days will be required for the cytopathic effect to appear and with the slower growing viruses several weeks may elapse before the virus is found to be present. Virus isolation does therefore tend to be a relatively slow method of diagnosis.

SEROLOGY

An alternative approach to the diagnosis of virus disease in the surviving animal is to demonstrate a high or rising antibody titre to a particular virus. With some diseases, the antibody titre following recovery from natural infection is very much higher than that produced by vaccination, so the demonstration of a high titre is often taken as presumptive evidence of recent infection. However, unless the animal is a puppy or kitten, it is always possible that the antibody has been present for some considerable time and is not related to the current illness. Ideally, therefore, paired blood samples, i.e. an acute phase sample and a convalescent sample collected two weeks later, should always be submitted for examination. Even this procedure may sometimes fail to provide a definite result because the animal may have been infected for longer than supposed and the titre may already have reached its peak when the first blood sample was collected. This often applies to cases of canine distemper and an additional problem with this disease is that immuno-suppression often occurs so the antibody titre never does rise. Conversely, with canine parvovirus and canine adenovirus infections, antibody is produced very rapidly and a fairly high titre may already be present when the first blood sample is taken; one or two days delay in collecting the first blood sample may well be crucial.

The choice of serological test to be employed in diagnostic work is essentially pragmatic. Canine parvovirus agglutinates pig red cells and since haemagglutination is a simple procedure and one providing a rapid result, haemagglutination-inhibition is much preferable to neutralisation which is much more labour intensive, more expensive and much slower in producing results. With canine adenovirus and canine parainfluenza virus, on the other hand, neutralisation is preferred because it gives more consistent and easily interpretable results than haemagglutination-inhibition. In due course, the enzyme-linked immuno-sorbent assay (ELISA test) may well replace these older procedures. It is, of course, already in use for feline leukaemia but for the detection of antigen rather than antibody. Like the haemagglutination-inhibition test, the ELISA test will give the results within a few hours. Neutralisation, on the other hand, will require up to five days.

When serology is required as a check that an animal has responded to vaccination, it is important to remember that it is only the neutralisation test that directly demonstrates the presence of **protective** antibody. The immune response to virus infection results in the production of antibodies to several different virus antigens. However, it is generally only one of these antibodies that is capable of neutralising the virus and hence protecting the animal. The ELISA test will not discriminate between protective and non-protective antibodies and therefore, unless specially adapted, cannot be used as proof that an animal is actually protected against a given virus infection. In some infections, neutralising antibody will also inhibit haemagglutination; the haemagglutination-inhibition test can then be used to demonstrate, albeit indirectly, protective antibody. Canine parvovirus falls essentially into this category.

In testing the immune status of an animal and in serological work generally, it must not be thought that the results obtained in one type of test are comparable with those obtained in another. Each type of test has its own threshold sensitivity and even when a supposedly identical test is carried out in two different laboratories, there will be factors which result in a difference in sensitivity.

One last word of advice: Since virological facilities and expertise available to the practitioner are strictly limited, when in doubt it is always best to telephone a laboratory, discuss your problem with an appropriate person there and find out what the laboratory can do to help. This may avoid the wastage of a lot of time and effort in sending material to a laboratory which cannot handle it or in submitting unsuitable specimens to a laboratory which does have the necessary facilities.

SAMPLING PROCEDURES

SELECTION OF SAMPLES

It is important to remember that the differences between the various virus families are just as great as those existing between different types of vertebrate. What applies to one particular virus does not therefore, necessarily apply to another. Selection of the most suitable material for submission to the virus laboratory therefore depends partly on the characteristics of the virus itself and partly on those of the disease it produces. If, for example, as in the case of canine distemper, immuno-suppression occurs, the serological response will be poor so that the submission of a blood sample for the determination of its antibody titre is unlikely to be rewarding. With canine adenovirus infection, on the other hand, there is no immuno-suppression and recovery is accompanied by the rapid production of specific antibody to a very high titre indeed.

If an animal dies or is euthanised on humane grounds, there is a wide choice of material for submission to the virus laboratory. Unless one is dealing with a severe but superficial infection, as for example with respiratory virus infection in young kittens, there is absolutely no point in taking swabs — which can only absorb a limited amount of virus — when tissues possibly containing high titres of virus are available. Similarly, there is nothing to be gained by submitting a blood sample for serology and incinerating the carcase and organs which may be rich in virus. The choice of organs depends upon recognition of lesions, knowledge of the exact target organs of the virus and the stage reached in the disease process. It should always be borne in mind that the longer the animal has been infected, the greater the influence of the immune response and other factors in modifying the distribution and quantity of virus present.

With diseases such as kennel cough, in which the mortality rate is negligible, or with individual animals which manage to recover from the more serious systemic diseases, tissues will not be available, so an alternative strategy must be sought. Depending upon the actual target sites, easily procurable excretions such as faeces and urine may contain virus but they are less than ideal for inoculation into delicate cell-cultures. That is one reason why it is much easier to demonstrate parvovirus haemagglutinin in faeces samples than to isolate the virus contained in them. In many diseases the animal is viraemic but, with the obvious exceptions of feline leukaemia and feline immunosuppression virus infections, the duration of viraemia is often limited to a few days only so that attempted virus isolation from a blood sample may be unsuccessful. False negative results can therefore easily occur. The pharynx and tonsils are one of the most important portals of entry in many virus diseases and virus may be present at these sites for some considerable time after infection, generally until eliminated by the immune response. The submission of pharyngeal swabs may therefore sometimes permit virus isolation, particularly in the case of the respiratory infections of both dog and cat.

Since many viruses are very labile structures, easily inactivated by heat at normal environment temperatures and, in some cases, by drying, all swabs for virus isolation should be immersed in virus transport medium. This is a liquid tissue culture medium containing serum proteins which exert a protective effect on the virus. It also contains antibiotics which control bacteria in the sample and hence prevent not only damage to the virus itself but damage to the cell-cultures when they are inoculated with the virus-containing transport medium. Before use, the swab should be immersed in the transport medium so that any virus picked up tends to lie on or near the surface rather than be absorbed into the interior of the swab. The use of gelatinous or charcoal bacteriological transport media is quite counter-productive because there is no easy way of getting the virus out of these substances and into the cell culture.

COLLECTION OF SAMPLES

Most samples will contain biological materials which are sensitive and readily broken down. Tissues intended for immuno-fluorescence or virus isolation decompose rapidly, especially in anaerobic conditions. Viruses are very susceptible to thermal inactivation and bacteria or fungi present in swabs and other material may multiply in these specimens to render them quite unsuitable for inoculation into cell-culture. For this reason, serum and tissue samples should always be collected aseptically and swabs and fresh tissue for virus isolation should always be transported in virus transport medium. All samples should be refrigerated between collection and postage.

All samples should be accompanied by a history which should include such details as the name of the owner, the sex, breed and age of the animal and a brief description of the clinical signs or post-mortem lesions found. Where relevant, the vaccination history should be given and it is very important that the commercial brand of vaccine used be clearly stated.

Canine Distemper

Fatal cases. Virus isolation is generally not a practical proposition. Small portions (about 1 cm cube) of lung, thymus, spleen, retropharyngeal lymph node, urinary bladder, renal pelvis, ileum, cerebellum and hindbrain stem, should be submitted in 10% formalin for histopathological examination. In the hands of an experienced pathologist, it is often possible to reach a diagnosis on histopathological criteria, provided all of the above range of tissues have been submitted. If immunofluorescence tests are available (telephone laboratory to ascertain), small pieces of lymphoid tissue, lungs and hindbrain should be submitted fresh.

Surviving animal. Definitive diagnosis of distemper in the living animal is extremely difficult and therefore only occasionally possible. Virus isolation from swabs or blood is not a practical proposition. Examination of conjunctival smears, whether by immunofluorescence or by conventional staining, is insensitive and difficult to interpret. In some cases, it is possible to demonstrate a significant rise in antibody titre in paired blood samples. Two samples (2 — 5 ml each) of clotted blood should be collected at an interval of two weeks. A sample of cerebrospinal fluid (1 ml should suffice) may permit the demonstration of specific antibody in some cases of canine distemper virus — related encephalitis, particularly those presenting as a primary encephalitis.

There is a test, performed on urine, offered by some commercial laboratories but the author has no direct experience of this.

For the evaluation of the immune status of a vaccinated dog, 2 — 5 ml of clotted blood should be submitted.

Canine Parvovirus Infection

Fatal cases. Histopathology of the intestines and lymphoid tissues is the most reliable method of confirming parvovirus enteritis. A small piece of the duodenum and jejunum, together with similar sized portions of different levels of the ileum, should be placed in 10% formol saline. Pieces of thymus (if present) and mesenteric lymph node should also be included.

In the rare event of a puppy dying of parvovirus myocarditis, histopathology of the heart muscle is diagnostic.

Surviving animals. In clinically affected animals, both faeces (5 ml) and clotted blood (5 ml) samples should be submitted for diagnosis.

For the evaluation of immunity in a vaccinated dog, 2 — 5 ml of clotted blood should be sent to the laboratory.

Infectious Canine Hepatitus

Fatal cases. A small block of liver, about 1 cm cube, should be submitted in virus transport medium for virus isolation. A similar sized block of tissue, together with hepatic or mesenteric lymph node, spleen and kidney, should be placed in 10% formol saline for histopathology.

Surviving animals. Two clotted blood samples, each of 2 — 5 ml, should be collected for serology, the first when the dog is initially presented and the second a fortnight later.

Canine Herpesvirus Infection

Neonatal puppies. Small blocks of liver, renal cortex, lung and spleen should be submitted in virus transport medium for virus isolation.

Adult carriers. There is no proven serological test for antibody to canine herpesvirus. Demonstration of past infection, let alone the carrier state, is therefore impossible by current serological methods.

The author has failed to isolate the virus from a single one of the numerous vaginal and prepucial swabs he has received. There is only one report in the literature of virus isolation from the genital tract of non-pregnant/non-nursing bitches and that was when vesicular lesions were present on the external genitalia.

Kennel Cough

Canine parainfluenza virus, both serotypes of canine adenovirus and, more rarely, canine herpesvirus are known to be able to cause respiratory disease. All three viruses can readily be isolated in cell-culture. It is clear however, that some outbreaks of respiratory disease can occur without the involvement of any of these viruses. It is possible that another virus is involved in some outbreaks, one which does not grow under the conditions employed for the isolation of, for example, adenovirus.

Nasal and tonsillar swabs in virus transport medium should be submitted for virus isolation. Swabs should be taken from recent arrivals in the kennels as well as from clinically affected dogs.

Paired blood samples (2 — 5 ml of clotted blood) can be submitted to the laboratory for adenovirus and parainfluenza virus serology. If parainfluenza is suspected, it may be best to extend the interval between the samples to three weeks, as serum antibody is slow to develop in this infection.

Infectious Diarrohea of the Dog

When diarrhoea occurs in kennels but is unlikely to be of dietary origin or caused by recognised viral or bacterial pathogens, it may be possible, by special arrangement, to have faeces samples examined for the presence of canine calicivirus, canine coronavirus and canine rotavirus. This is done by electron microscopy, though the calicivirus can also be isolated in cell culture under appropriate conditions. Samples should consist of 5 — 10 ml of fresh faeces.

Feline Respiratory Virus Infections

Feline calicivirus and feline herpesvirus both grow readily in feline cell-cultures. The herpesvirus is a labile structure which is quickly inactivated under dry conditions. For virus isolation, tonsillar swabs should be taken and submitted to the laboratory in virus transport medium to prevent dehydration.

Feline Panleucopaenia

Fatal cases. Exactly the same samples are required for this as for the diagnosis of canine parvovirus infection. The virus agglutinates red cells under rather narrow conditions. The main approach is, therefore, the histopathological one.

Surviving animals. The most convenient method is by serology, antibody titres in clotted blood (1 — 2 ml) samples being measured by an haemagglutination-inhibition test using canine parvovirus.

Feline Infectious Peritonitis

Many coronaviruses are notoriously difficult to grow in cell-culture. At present, therefore, immunofluorescence is used to measure the titre of antibody in the serum of suspected cases. 1 — 2 ml of clotted blood or 1 ml of ascitic fluid should be submitted for serology.

Feline Leukaemia

The object is to demonstrate viraemia. Initially, the blood is screened for antigen by a commercial ELISA test. Positive results are then confirmed by virus isolation in cell-culture. For this purpose 1 — 2 ml of **heparinised** blood is required. The use of EDTA to prevent the blood from clotting renders the sample useless for virus isolation as the EDTA effectively destroys the cell culture.

It may sometimes be desirable to check serologically that a cat has recovered from infection and is therefore likely to be resistant to reinfection. This is done by the demostration of virus neutralising antibody in a sample of 1 — 2 ml of clotted blood.

Feline T-Lymphotropic Lentivirus (FLTV) now called
Feline Immunosuppression Virus (FIV)

Virus isolation from the blood is difficult and generally not a practical proposition. Since viraemia is usually correlated with the presence of antibody, diagnosis can be confirmed by the demonstration of antibody by a commercial ELISA test. For this purpose 1 — 2 ml of clotted or heparinised blood should be submitted. The use of heparinised blood is an exception to the important rule that **serum** (extracted from **clotted** blood) is required for **serology**. In this instance, heparinised blood is advantageous, not only because the plasma obtained from it is suitable for ELISA tests, but also because it provides appropriate material for virus isolation, should this be thought worth while.

INTERPRETATION OF RESULTS

In general, the isolation of a virus is highly significant diagnostically but it should be borne in mind that some viruses, e.g reoviruses, are of very low pathogenicity while others, though highly pathogenic in non-immune animals, can produce persistent infections and may therefore still be present in certain tissues many months after the initial infection. Conversely, negative results obtained on attempted virus isolation do not necessarily rule out a diagnosis. This applies specially to the more acute infections. Respiratory virus infection — but not secondary bacterial infection — may often have been eliminated by the time the first swab is taken. With feline leukaemia, on the other hand, the persistent viraemia means that the probability of isolating virus from a single blood sample is very high, the probability of a false negative result therefore being correspondingly low. This assumes, of course, that the correct material is submitted in the prescribed manner.

Interpretation of serological data tends to be more complex, though if a statistically significant increase (usually greater than fourfold) in antibody titre can be demonstrated in paired blood samples, this is generally regarded as diagnostic. However, even in the presence of an immune response, it is not always possible to demonstrate a rising titre. Antibody is produced more quickly to some virus infections than to others. In some instances, therefore, the titre will already be at or near its peak when the first sample is taken. In others, e.g. canine parainfluenza virus infection, antibody titres may still be low at the time the second sample is collected. The submission of single, rather than paired, blood samples obviously imposes further limits to the extent to which a result can be interpreted for diagnostic purposes. Some useful information can, however, often be obtained.

SPECIFIC DISEASE ASSESSMENT

Canine Distemper.

The essential point to grasp is that the dog with obvious clinical distemper is affected in that way because the virus has caused immunosuppression and cannot therefore be eliminated. This means that the antibody titre will be low, not high. Typical neutralising antibody titres lie in the range 24 — 128. Conversely, dogs which recover rapidly, having shown little or no clinical signs of the disease have titres of 16384 or more. So, although a titre of 90 is typical of clinical distemper, it is not diagnostic because a disease cannot be diagnosed on negative criteria. A low titre is a bad prognostic sign, but because the cell-mediated immune response plays a major role in the recovery process, dogs with antibody titres as low as 128 do sometimes make an apparently complete recovery. Conversely, some dogs with much higher antibody titres occasionally succumb to neurological disease. Immunosuppression is often partial so that some clinical signs and moderate titres of antibody are produced.

Neutralising antibody found in a single blood sample may have been present for weeks, months or years. Unless, therefore, one is dealing with a puppy, the antibody cannot be related to **recent** infection. Paired blood samples are therefore essential for diagnosis though, because of immunosuppression, the titre may fail to rise, so that in only a proportion of cases is it possible to obtain a diagnosis in this way. In a minority of cases of nervous distemper, it is possible to demonstrate antibody in the cerebro-spinal fluid. This is diagnostic because there is no antibody in the fluid of the normal solidly immune dog.

If one is dealing with apparent breakdowns in immunity in vaccinated dogs, it is important to realise that the range of antibody titre produced by vaccination corresponds exactly to that resulting from natural infection, i.e. from 24 to >32768, though good vaccines should produce a titre of 128 at the very least. Any antibody demonstrated in such cases could therefore be due either to vaccination or to natural infection. If, however, antibody is absent or present to a very low titre, vaccination has clearly been ineffective and the owner may have a legitimate claim against the manufacturer of the vaccine.

Canine Parvovirus Infection

Anitbody appears very rapidly in the blood following infection. Antibody reaching the intestinal lumen eliminates virus from the intestine, the virus initially being complexed with the antibody. Complexed virus is not readily detectable by either haemagglutination or ELISA tests and this can lead to false negative results with both tests. However, such animals will generally have very high antibody titres, >2048 in the haemagglutination-inhibition test. Titres of this magnitude can be produced by vaccination with live canine parvovirus vaccine but whereas some vaccines will do this in 80 — 90 per cent of recipients, others will do it in only about one third of innoculated animals, the titres of many lying in the range of 64 — 512. These moderate titres are readily distinguished from those of naturally-infected dogs. Inactivated vaccines also produce low or moderate antibody titres so again there is no problem in distinguishing a vaccinal titre from one resulting from natural exposure.

Canine Adenovirus Infection

There is a very close antigenic relationship between the two canine adenoviruses. After a second exposure to either type of virus, a dog will possess antibody which has approximately the same titre to each type. It can, therefore, be difficult to distinguish infection with one type from infection with the other by serological means. A dog recovering from infectious canine hepatitis will have a high antibody titre to the heterologous virus (e.g. 16384) and although this may not be as high as its titre to the homologous virus, it is generally well above the titres produced by vaccination, which rarely exceed 4096 and are generally lower (range 64 — 4096).

Canine Parainfluenza Virus

Vaccination by the subcutaneous route generally fails to elicit neutralising antibody in demonstrable amounts but titres of up to 64 are occasionally found. Vaccination by the intranasal route results in the production not only of local antibody but also serum antibody, serum titres of 256 — 4096 being detectable by the neutralisation test. Following exposure to natural infection, neutralising antibody titres of 2048 — 16384 or more are produced though the immune response does seem to be slower than in systemic virus infections.

Feline Infectious Peritonitis

It is impossible to distinguish serologically between the coronavirus which causes feline infectious peritonitis and other feline coronaviruses which cause enteritis or asymptomatic infections. Interpretation of the serological titre must always be made with full regard to the clinical signs and general circumstances of the case.

Suspected case. In cases of the effusive form of the disease, the titre can fall to a very low level in the terminal stages. It is thought that the antibody in these moribund cats is bound up in complexes and therefore unavailable for the test. However, in the vast majority of cases, the absence of a titre indicates that the cat does not have the disease. Conversely, if there is a titre of any level in a sick cat, feline infectious peritonitis must be suspected. Titres often rise to >1280 but if the titre is lower, it may be useful to take a second blood sample two to three weeks later to see if the titre is rising. In effusive cases with severe ascites, a titre can be regarded as sufficient grounds for euthanasia but in other cases a definitive diagnosis can only be made by histopathology.

Clinically healthy in-contact cat. If no antibody is demonstrable, infection can generally be ruled out. With titres of up to 20, the cat will probably be all right. If, however, the titre is over 20, another blood sample should be submitted 6 — 8 weeks later. If this shows the titre to be rising, either the cat is developing the disease or it is still in contact with one shedding the virus. If the titre is falling, the cat is no longer exposed to coronaviruses and will not develop the disease. Only about 10% of cats that seroconvert go on to develop the disease. There is no correlation between the height of the titre and the likelihood that the cat will develop the disease.

Screening for mating. In a cattery which is free of coronavirus, only those cats which are entirely free of antibody can safely be admitted.

CHAPTER 10

IMMUNOLOGICAL TECHNIQUES

D. R. E. Jones M.Sc., Ph.D., F.I.M.L.S.

INTRODUCTION

Protection of the body's internal environment against invasion from without is mediated via a lymphoreticular network — the immune system. This diffuse organ monitors the identity of the body: its basic constituents are lymphocytes and antibodies, which recognise both foreign molecules (antigens) and one another. A complex network of control factors exists to regulate the immune response, indicating a number of ways in which it may become abnormal. Thus, disorders of the immune system may result in a failure of self-recognition (autoimmune diseases), an inadequate response to antigenic challenge (immunodeficiency diseases) or abnormal uncontrolled responses (immunoproliferative diseases). Consequently, immunological techniques have become established in veterinary clinical laboratories — not only providing sensitive and unequivocal diagnostic tests but also giving an insight into the aetiology and pathogenesis of many disease processes.

Many immunological assays require 'hands on' demonstration by personnel having experience of the techniques and principles involved. Often, results are comparative and a number of controls must be run simultaneously — necessitating access to (stored) samples which will give predictable results. Indeed, in some circumstances, more controls than tests need to be included in an assay procedure. Such techniques are unsuitable for most practice laboratories and consequently in many of the areas described, only the technique principles will be given. Comments on the various approaches which can be used will also be given where applicable. No techniques requiring, for example, skin biopsies are described. It is felt that the processing of such material for immunoassay will remain in the specialised laboratory at least for the present.

SAMPLE COLLECTION

With the exception of some diagnostic tests for autoimmune haemolytic anaemia, all the assays described can be performed on a sample of clotted blood (i.e. on serum). This can be collected using any of the commonly available methods (vacutainers, monovettes or syringes). A clotted blood sample must be centrifuged (1500 x g : 10 minutes) to obtain cell-free serum, which is separated immediately.

Fresh blood will be required for the diagnosis of autoimmune haemolytic anaemia in order to demonstrate red blood cell-bound antibody/complement. Elution of bound antibody has been shown to occur gradually *in vitro* and this may lead to false negative results. The blood sample should be taken into acid citrate dextrose (ACD) solution or citrate phosphate dextrose (CPD) solution (1 volume anticoagulant to 4 volumes blood). Both ACD and CPD can be obtained from blood transfusion packs (they are used as anticoagulants for blood transfusion), or prepared sample tubes may be obtained from specialist diagnostic laboratories. A volume of 2.5 ml — 5.0 ml of sample is sufficient for most screening tests. EDTA blood samples have been used to provide red cells for autoimmune haemolytic anaemia diagnosis but false negative results can occur with this anticoagulant, particularly when haemolysis is observed in the sample tube. Samples (both whole blood and unseparated clotted blood) must not be stored in a refrigerator. It is known than complement components and non-pathological antibodies ('normal cold antibodies') can be absorbed on to the red blood cells (RBC) at low temperatures. Thus, red blood cells (RBC) subsequently tested may give a false positive result whereas separated serum may have been depleted of complement components. Separated serum may be sent through the post for some of the autoimmune haemolytic anaemia tests described.

LABORATORY METHODS AND INTERPRETATION

AUTOIMMUNE DISEASES

Autoimmune haemolytic anaemia (AHA)

A haemolytic anaemia is defined as any condition which results in a reduced red blood cell (RBC) life span. The presence of antibody(ies) directed against 'self' RBC antigen(s) is the pertinent feature of AHA. Diagnostic criteria for the condition involve the demonstration of antibody which either coats autologous RBC *in vivo* or which can be detected in the serum. Some of these autoantibodies are able to activate complement. Hence complement components (notably component C3) may also be detected on the RBC. Thus, laboratory diagnostic tests must be employed to determine the presence of autoantibody and/or complement (C3) on the RBC. Alternatively, the presence of serum antibody(ies) may be used in the diagnosis.

The classical description of AHA involves sudden onset of anaemia, the blood picture indicating a marked regeneration. However, it is now appreciated that it can present with a complete spectrum of haematological findings from a non-regenerative (aplastic) picture through a normocytic, normochromic anaemia to the more commonly described regenerative response. Thus an anaemia, of whatever type, should be investigated for a possible immune-mediated aetiology if no obvious underlying cause can be demonstrated. It should be noted also that AHA can occur secondary to a variety of disease processes, particularly neoplastic conditions and especially those involving haematological malignancy.

Before use in any diagnostic tests for autoimmune haemolytic anaemia (i.e. serological tests), RBC must be thoroughly washed in order to remove all traces of plasma proteins which could inhibit subsequent immunological reactions. This washing procedure should be carried out using isotonic phosphate buffered saline (PBS), which is less likely than saline to produce haemolysis of the relatively fragile red cells from cases of AHA.

1. Centrifuge the anticoagulated blood sample : 1500 x g for 3 minutes is sufficient.
2. Remove the supernatant (taking note of any haemolysis, if present). At this stage the buffy coat (containing white blood cells and platelets) should also be removed, using a Pasteur pipette. Wherever possible, it is advisable to connect the Pasteur pipette to a suction pump and to remove the supernatant and buffy coat in one operation. White cells and platelets remaining in the red cell fraction can subsequently form spontaneous clumps which may be mistaken for agglutination under some circumstances.
3. Place an aliquot of red cells in an appropriate centrifuge tube (a plastic disposable tube is adequate). Add PBS to give a final ratio of (minimum) 9 volumes PBS to 1 volume of cells (small samples or profound anaemia will necessitate adjustment of these amounts). Mix well by inverting the tube several times.
4. Centrifuge : 1500 x g for approximately 2 minutes is sufficient. Remove supernatant. (Use a Pasteur pipette — preferably connected to a suction pump — to avoids loss of RBC which would inevitably occur if the tube was inverted).
5. Repeat the wash procedure : a total of 6 times in all. After each centrifugation step, the RBC should remain 'packed' in the bottom of the tube when the supernatant wash solution has been discarded.
6. After the final wash (and removal of the supernatant) the RBC must be re-suspended in PBS for use. The exact concentration of RBC will be dependent on the test system being used. A reasonably accurate RBC suspension can be obtained based on the original volume of packed cells used. Thus, if the original volume of centrifuged RBC was approximately 1 ml, addition of 9 ml PBS will provide

a 10% cell suspension. It is advisable to make up a 10% cell suspension, in any case, after washing and to use this as a 'stock'. Never keep packed washed RBC without any diluent — they will quickly haemolyse.

Papain Test.

This is a simple **screening** test for AHA. It has been used in canine diagnosis for a number of years and there is some evidence to suggest that it may be useful for the diagnosis of feline AHA.

The test requires the presence of RBC autoantibody(ies) in the serum of the patient. The proteolytic enzyme papain alters the surface properties of RBC so that agglutination (by these autoantibodies) will be enhanced. The papain solution used in the test is partially inactivated (to ensure that it cannot haemolyse RBC), a procedure normally carried out at a specialised laboratory.

Procedure

1. Incubate 100 μl washed packed patient RBC with 100 ul of activated papain solution (diluted 1/10 in isotonic PBS at pH 7.2) at 37°C for 15 minutes.

2. Wash RBC twice in PBS (to remove excess papain).

3. Resuspend washed RBC as a 5% suspension in PBS.

4. Add 1 volume of autologous serum to an equal volume of 5% papain-treated RBC. (Conveniently : 2 drops serum + 2 drops 5% RBC delivered via a standard ('short form') Pasteur pipette.)

5. Incubate at room temperature for 1 hour.

6. Inspect the tube for the presence of RBC agglutination.

For this (and other agglutination procedures) it is convenient to use disposable 10 mm x 75 mm plastic test tubes. It is not advisable to re-use such tubes because traces of serum protein may adhere to the plastic and inhibit agglutination reactions in subsequent tests. Agglutination is detected by gently tilting the tube from the vertical to the horizontal, allowing the button of RBC to run towards the mouth of the tube. Examination is made easier by employing direct light against a white background and by using a magnifying lens. Agglutination, if present, may be graded — from C (complete : all RBC agglutinated) through V (visual : a few large clumps of RBC) to + +, +, (+) and wk (weak). The latter two categories need to be confirmed by low power microscopy since they involve clumps of 4 — 6 RBC. In practice it is usually only necessary to distinguish between positive and negative because grades of agglutination have doubtful clinical relevance.

As a negative control, 1 volume of 5% papain-treated RBC is incubated with 1 volume of PBS. For a positive control, it is recommended that serum obtained from an animal with proven AHA is stored frozen (-20°C) in small aliquots and used in the papain test, alongside patient samples. Serum obtained from cases demonstrated to have AHA will agglutinate papain-treated RBC from all animals of the same species. Thus, it is feasible that the papain test can be carried out using patient serum incubated with a 'panel' of normal papain-treated RBC (in practice, 6 animals would suffice). However, the role of (non-pathological) naturally-occurring blood group antibodies in these 'indirect' reactions remains to be elucidated, so that the results would need to be interpreted with caution.

Coombs Test

For an unequivocal diagnosis of AHA, the presence of autoantibody and/or complement (as C3) must be demonstrated on the patient's RBC. The Coombs test (antiglobulin test) relies on the agglutination of these coated RBC by a specific antiserum (usually raised in rabbits) which will detect immunoglobulin and complement. In the direct Coombs test (direct antiglobulin test: DAT), washed RBC are incubated with the antiserum and if positive (i.e. coated with autoantibody and/or complement) agglutination will occur. In the indirect Coombs test (indirect antiglobulin test: IAT) RBC which are negative in the DAT are first incubated with autologous serum (to allow uptake of autoantibody) before being washed and re-incubated with the specific antiserum. Thus, if autoantibody (and complement) coat the RBC after the initial serum incubation phase, agglutination will be noted when the cells are subsequently exposed to a specific antiserum.

The antiglobulin reagent (Coombs reagent) used is subject to quality control procedures to ensure that it will detect IgG and C3. It is difficult to detect IgM on RBC using agglutination tests. However, because most IgM antibodies will fix C3, it is only necessary to have anti C3 (and anti IgG) activity in the reagent. Both IgG and IgM have been shown to coat RBC in AHA. In practice, a more reliable Coombs reagent can be produced from a 'cocktail' made up of monospecific anti IgG + monospecific anti C3, rather than the more traditional 'anti globulin' often described. In a specialised serology laboratory, the two specific antisera would be used individually (along with a specific anti IgM, if available) — on separate aliquots of the same RBC. In this way, data would be obtained on the amount and type of autoantibody present and whether or not it can activate complement. In a Coombs test, the autoantibody/complement is titrated against dilutions of the reagent. The antiserum is diluted in PBS (usually to at least 1/1024) for use.

Procedure (a) DAT.

1. Doubling dilutions of antiserum are prepared in PBS, using 10 mm x 75 mm plastic test tubes. One volume (= 2 drops dispensed from a Pasteur pipette) of each dilution is then transferred to further series of 10 mm x 75 mm tubes for use.

2. Add an equal volume of a 10% suspension of RBC to each tube. Mix by gentle agitation.

3. Incubate at 37°C for 1 hour.

4. Examine each tube for agglutination (as described above). The titre recorded is the last tube in which agglutination is noted.

For a negative control, use PBS in place of Coombs reagent in a further tube. The production of a positive control for the Coombs test involves the use of RBC which have been coated with known amounts of immunoglobulin(s) and/or C3. This procedure would normally only be carried out in a specialist laboratory. If no positive control is employed to check the efficacy of the reagent, a negative result must be interpreted with caution.

Autoagglutination (spontaneous clumping of RBC in the sample tube or in diluent) is sometimes noted in AHA. The appearance of this phenomenon in the negative control tube will negate results from a Coombs test. Autoagglutination, not dispersed by washing the RBC, is highly suggestive of AHA.

Procedure (b) IAT.

The indirect Coombs test is insensitive when applied to canine blood samples and papain-treated RBC are required to ensure autoantibody uptake from serum. No information is currently available regarding the use of an IAT in feline medicine and this field requires further study. Thus the IAT, when applied to the diagnosis of canine AHA, is more correctly termed the 'enzyme indirect antiglobulin test' (EIAT).

1. 1 volume of washed, **packed,** papain-treated RBC is incubated with 4 volumes of autologous serum, at room temperature for 90 minutes. The tube should be gently agitated occasionally to resuspend the cells. 100 μl of RBC + 400 μl of serum will suffice for this test.

2. Centrifuge the tube : approximately 1000 x g for 30 seconds. Remove supernatant.

3. Wash the RBC 6 times in PBS. Ice-cold PBS should be used to ensure that no antibody taken up is eluted off the RBC in the washing procedure.

4. Resuspend washed RBC at a 10% concentration in PBS.

5. The RBC are then put up against doubling dilutions of antiserum exactly as described for the DAT. Incubate at 37°C for 1 hour.

6. Examine each tube for agglutination.

A negative control must be included i.e. a tube containing washed sensitised RBC (as above) + PBS. A positive control should also be included — as described for the DAT.

In theory it is possible to carry out the EIAT using serum incubated with washed RBC from a normal animal (preferably, a 'panel' of normal RBC — from at least six animals). However, false positive reactions may be encountered due to naturally-occurring (blood group) antibodies.

A direct and indirect Coombs test can also be carried out using an enzyme-linked immunosorbent assay (ELISA). The technique has been successfully applied to canine AHA. Washed RBC are incubated with specific antisera (rabbit anti dog IgG, rabbit anti dog IgM and rabbit anti dog C3) in a 96 well microtitre plate. The cells are then washed *(in situ)* and a second antibody added : sheep anti rabbit IgG conjugated to an enzyme, alkaline phosphatase. The second antibody will combine with any anti IgG, anti IgM or anti C3 which has coated the RBC subsequent to the intitial incubation phase. After a further incubation period followed by washing, the cells are incubated with a specific substrate. This substrate (p-nitrophenyl phosphate) is converted to a yellow product by the conjugated enzyme. Thus, the intensity of the coloured reaction product — measured in a spectrophotometer (MicroELISA reader) — is proportional to the amount of conjugate and therefore first antibody, adhering to the RBC. The technique gives an objective assessment of RBC sensitisation in AHA (not always possible when the degree of agglutination is being measured by the naked eye) and enables small volumes of sample material to be used. 500 μl of a 2% suspension is sufficient for assay of cell-bound IgG, IgM and C3. However, relatively specialised equipment is required which places the technique outside the scope of a small practice laboratory. It is likely that innovative equipment design in the future will alter this situation. ELISA methodology can be used to detect a variety of serum antibodies, in a number of disease processes. An outline of the basic technique is given in Figure 10.1.

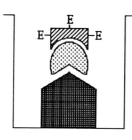

1. Antigen absorbed on to microtitre plate.
(in the Coombs test antigen = RBC)

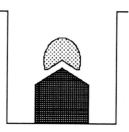

2. Add specific antibody
Antibody attaches to antigen

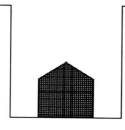

3. Add enzyme-labelled antibody

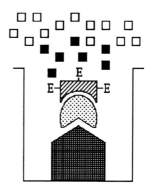

4. Add substrate.
Amount hydrolysed by enzyme = amount of antigen present
Read colour in spectrophotometer.

Figure 10.1
Principle of the Enzyme-linked Immunosorbent Assay

Immune-mediated thrombocytopenic purpura (IMPT)

IMTP is caused by a reduction in platelet (= thrombocyte) numbers below that required for the maintenance of vascular integrity and a normal bleeding time (haemostasis). Platelets are sensitised by an IgG autoantibody and demonstration of this antibody in laboratory assays is the essential diagnostic criterion.

A number of techniques have been employed to detect anti platelet antibody in suspected IMTP, with varying degrees of success.

1. **Direct Agglutination.** A suspension of platelets (taken from a normal 'control' animal) in PBS is incubated with test serum. This test gives equivocal results due to the frequently observed non-specific platelet clumping often seen *in vitro* and which can occur irrespective of the presence of antibody.

2. **Direct Immunofluorescence.** A rabbit anti IgG conjugated to a fluorescent label (fluorescein isothiocyanate — FITC) is used directly on a bone marrow biopsy smear, prepared from an animal with suspected IMTP. Fluorescence on megakaryocytes can be demonstrated , in some cases, when (auto)antibody has coated these platelet-precursor cells. In practice, megakaryocytes may not always be found in bone marrow biopsy smears prepared from cases with thrombocytopenia or the cells may be small and morphologically indistinct.

3. **Antiglobulin Consumption Test.** A direct antiglobulin test (DAT; Coombs test) is prepared. RBC coated with a known amount of IgG are used and a specific rabbit anti IgG employed as the agglutinating reagent. The DAT should give a significant titre (ideally > 1/128). Serum from a case with suspected IMTP is added to the test system (in a parallel row of tubes) and a reduction in the titre will occur if an IgG autoantibody is present (and which interferes with the DAT reaction). Meticulously prepared controls are needed. These should include normal serum, diluent (PBS only) as negative controls and serum from a case of confirmed IMTP (known to contain the IgG autoantibody) as a positive control. In practice, the test is difficult to standardise and gives variable results in both negative and positive control tubes.

4. **Platelet Factor 3 (PF3) Test.** The PF3 test has been used for the diagnosis of canine IMTP. The test relies on the release of PF3 from platelets as a result of exposure to autoantibody directed against the platelet membrane. Platelet-rich plasma (PRP) from a normal animal is incubated with normal globulin and the patient's globulin (prepared from serum by dialysis) in the presence of Contact Product (activated clotting factors XI and XII). If anti platelet antibody is present in the globulin fraction of the test serum, the clotting time of the PRP (initiated by the addition of 0.025M calcium chloride) is shortened as compared with the normal control. However, many cases of suspected IMTP fail to show a positive PF3 test. It is important, also, that all samples of PRP used contain the same relative numbers of platelets. This requires an accurate platelet counting method, employing sophisticated electronic counting equipment.

    It is likely that ELISA procedures, currently being used for the measurement of membrane-bound platelet IgG in human serology, will be adapted for use in small animal diagnostic medicine.

    It has not been ascertained to what extent (if any) the presence of (non-pathological) alloantibodies might influence the results of the **indirect** tests described. The whole field of platelet antibody testing poses many problems which remain to be resolved. In practice, IMTP often occurs concommitant with AHA, so that the presence of a positive DAT (or Papain Test) would be sufficient evidence for immune-mediated platelet depletion to be suspected.

Rheumatoid Arthritis (RA).

This disorder is often seen as a progressive polyarthritis affecting numerous organ systems. The most frequent site of injury is the synovial lining of the joints. In many cases of RA, an IgM antibody (rheumatoid factor — RF) can be demonstrated in the serum. RF has specificity for IgG and the circulating immune complexes which result appear to be involved in the inflammatory disease process, although a clear association is difficult to demonstrate. The presence of circulating RF is of diagnostic significance in RA patients, although some individuals with apparent RA may not have detectable RF. In the human disease, RF can be found in the joint fluid, where the titre tends to correlate with the severity of the lesions.

In canine serology, a modified Rose-Waaler test is employed for the measurement of RF in serum. A canine anti sheep erythrocyte serum is used to coat fresh, washed sheep RBC in a sub-agglutinating dose (i.e.

the cells are incubated with increasing dilutions of the antiserum to the point at which no agglutination takes place). After subsequent washing, these sensitised RBC will agglutinate when (test) serum containing IgG (i.e. RF) is introduced (Figure 10.2).

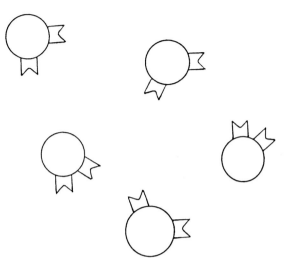

1. Sheep RBC coated with a sub-agglutinating dose of specific antibody (e.g. canine antisheep antibody : an IgG)

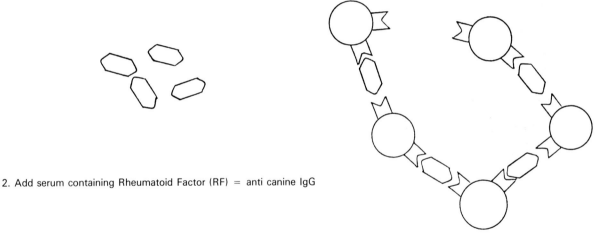

2. Add serum containing Rheumatoid Factor (RF) = anti canine IgG

3. Agglutination of RBC = RF positive

Figure 10.2
Principle of the Modified Rose-Waaler Test for Rheumatoid Factor.

Procedure.

1. Fresh patient's serum or serum stored at $-20°C$ is suitable. It must be heat inactivated at 56°C for 15 minutes in order to destroy complement.

2. Doubling dilutions of the serum are made in PBS (up to 1/512).

3. Equal volumes of the serum dilutions and 2% sensitised sheep RBC are mixed and incubated at 37°C for 1 hour.

4. Examine the tubes for agglutination.

An equivalent series of serum dilutions must also be incubated with unsensitised sheep RBC. A positive result is one in which the sensitised cells are agglutinated by at least a 4-fold greater dilution of serum compared with the unsensitised cells. Control tubes must be included, containing known positive and negative sera (for both the sensitised and the unsensitised cells).

Systemic Lupus Erythematosus (SLE)

SLE is a chronic multi-system disorder characterised by the presence of an anti-nuclear antibody (ANA) in the blood. Because the disorder can involve many organ systems it may present diagnostic problems. There may be simultaneous occurrence of two or more of the following disorders : autoimmune haemolytic anaemia, thrombocytopenic purpura, rheumatoid arthritis, immune complex glomerulonephritis, skin changes, hypergammaglobulinaemia. Various techniques have been employed for the laboratory diagnosis of SLE.

1. **LE Cell Test.** It has been stated that patients with SLE have an IgG anti-nuclear antibody which will react with nuclear material. Thus, the resulting homogeneous complex will be phagocytosed by granulocytes to form the characteristic LE cell. This is essentially an **in vitro** phenomenon and it can be visualised after granulocytes are traumatised. This is usually achieved by forcing clotted blood (which has been allowed to stand for 1—2 hours) through a sieve and centrifuging the resulting defibrinated material (10 minutes, 1500 x g). Smears are prepared from the buffy coat. These are stained using a standard (e.g. Leishman) technique. A typical LE cell is a granulocyte which has ingested homogeneous nuclear material. Thus, it appears with an eccentric nucleus and cytoplasm engorged with the ingested material. In practice, it is often difficult to identify LE cells unequivocally, due to the mass of degenerated cells and cellular debris present in such preparations. Various modifications to the technique have been described but all require disruption of granulocytes and often give ambiguous results. It has been noted that LE cells may be seen, using such techniques, in many pathological conditions and particularly after treatment with a wide range of drugs.

2. **Immunofluorescence Test (IFT).** 'Anti-nuclear antibody' (ANA) can be detected in serum using a fluorescein-labelled antibody specific for IgG. The nuclear material used in the test need not be of the same species as the test serum, since by definition, an antibody reacting with DNA will not necessarily be species-specific. The IFT uses frozen sections of rat liver as the substrate material. Slides with the substrate are incubated with serial dilutions of test serum, washed in PBS and then re-incubated with rabbit anti IgG (specific for the patient species) conjugated to FITC. Fluorescence of nuclear material in the section is visualised, after a final rinse and air drying, with a suitable microscope. Known negative and positive sera must be included as controls. Some fluorescence may be noted in negative control slides but a positive serum should give a reaction at a 2—4 fold higher dilution for an unequivocal result.

3. **Enzyme-Linked Immunosorbent Assay (ELISA).** DNA, obtained from calf thymus, is bound to wells in a microtitre plate and test serum added. Anti DNA (IgG) antibody, if present, will bind to the DNA preparation and can be measured after the addition of a second antibody (e.g. anti dog IgG conjugated to a peroxidase enzyme) followed by a specific substrate. The principle is essentially similar to that outlined in Figure 10.1. Negative and known positive sera must be included as controls. PBS is substituted for serum in a control for non-specific (i.e. background) activity. The antigen preparation used should be selected to allow detection of antibodies to double stranded (ds) DNA, which are regarded as specific for canine SLE.

4. **Radio-immunoassay (RIA).** This technique provides a sensitive and specific method for the detection of anti DNA antibodies in serum. In brief, isotope labelled (^{125}I) antigen is added to the test serum and the mixture treated with 50% saturated ammonium sulphate in order to precipitate immunoglobulins. The precipitate will contain radioactivity only if antigen-antibody complexes have formed. The amount of antibody can be estimated from the radioactivity detected. In the canine RIA system, precautions must be taken to prevent the high levels of non-specific DNA binding which can occur. Thus the serum must be heat-inactivated (60°C for 30 minutes) or dextran sulphate added. It has been suggested that similar procedures might be required for feline sera.

In practice, SLE may be accompanied by a Coombs positive anaemia, Rheumatoid Factor in serum and/or findings indicative of immune-mediated thrombocytopenia. Not all features of SLE may present simultaneously and unequivocal evidence of anti DNA antibodies (or anti nuclear antibody) may only be noted during clinical manifestations of the condition.

IMMUNODEFICIENCY DISEASES

An inadequate response to antigenic challenge may result from depletion of one (or more) of the gammaglobulins. Thus, the ability to produce a specific antibody response can be severely diminished. This type of immunodeficiency can be due to a lack of immunoglobulin (agammaglobulinaemia) or a reduction in levels of immunoglobulin (hypogammaglobulinaemia). These conditions may be the consequence of genetic transmission or they may be apparently acquired; i.e. through defective immunoglobulin synthesis, increased catabolism or excessive loss. In the latter category would be included renal disease or gastrointestinal disorders. Alternatively, there may be a selective immunoglobulin deficiency — e.g. IgA or IgG — a disorder termed dysgammaglobulinaemia. In addition, viral suppression may follow infection with any of several viruses; particularly those which localise in lymphocytes and cells of the reticuloendothelial system (e.g leukaemia viruses).

Investigation of gammaglobulin status as a possible contributory factor in an immunodeficiency state would require the following:

1. **Serum Protein Electrophoresis (SPE).** This technique serves as a screening test to give a general indication of the proteins present in serum, without specific characterisation. A drop of serum is applied to a suitable medium, in buffer, (cellulose acetate has been used extensively for this purpose, although agarose gel gives superior separation) and an electric current applied. The constituent proteins separate according to the charge on each molecule. They can be identified after the electrophoretic strip has been stained. The strip may be scanned using a densitometer, the percentage of each protein (according to intensity of staining) calculated and then related to the total protein concentration (in g/l) — see Figure 10.5. Gross changes may be apparent using this technique but more subtle fluctuations in individual proteins will require specific assays.

2. **Radial Immunodiffusion (RID).** This procedure is carried out in an agarose (1% in PBS) gel containing specific antiserum. RID is a specific quantitative technique which can be used to determine the amount of a specific immunoglobulin present in the serum. A specific antiserum with a high affinity for the protein (antigen) being assayed must be used. The antiserum is added to the agarose solution before the gel is poured — usually on to a glass plate. The gel sets on cooling and must be of a uniform thickness over the plate. Wells are punched in the gel, at an appropriate distance apart (determined by trial and error, initially). Test sera are pipetted into each well (volume required may be as little as 5 ul, depending on the test system/conditions), the plate is covered and placed in a humid chamber. Antigen, from each well, will diffuse into the gel to form an insoluble immunoprecipitate with the incorporated specific antiserum. The precipitate is trapped in the gel matrix, the diameter of the precitpitin ring thus formed being proportional to the concentration of antigen initially present. Room temperature is sufficient for RID. Diffusion will be more rapid at 37°C but the gel may dry out at this temperature. A series of standards must be included on each plate, to represent the range of antigen concentrations anticipated. The gel is incubated for 12 — 24 hours (ideally until the highest concentration standard has reached a plateau) and the ring diameters carefully measured (Figure 10.3). The precipitin rings may be visualised by holding the plate over a light source (or the gel can be stained if the patterns are to be preserved). Devices for reading the ring diameters are available from a number of laboratory suppliers. RID kits, which usually consist of standardised gels in sealed plastic containers, are available from commercial suppliers. Thus, serum IgG, IgM or IgA may be assayed in an RID system and the data obtained used to indicate the presence of a selective immunodeficiency.

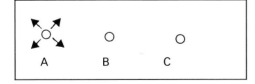

1. Antigen diffuses from wells into gel loaded with a highly specific antiserum

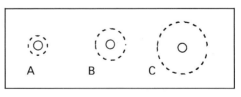

2. After completion of diffusion, the ring diameters are proportional to antigen concentration e.g. A = 2.0mg/ml B = 4.0mg/ml C = 10.0mg/ml

Figure 10.3
Radial Immunodiffusion (RID)

3. **Immunoelectrophoresis (IEP).** RID is a passive immunodiffusion technique — the antigen is allowed to diffuse freely into a gel matrix. IEP combines **active** separation of constituent serum proteins (electrophoresis) with **passive** diffusion of an antiserum against the separated proteins. The technique can separate serum into 20 or more fractions. IEP is principally a qualitative assay but as a screening procedure for the major classes of serum immunoglobulins it may be regarded as semiquantitative.

An agarose gel is prepared as for RID but **without** antiserum. The gel is allowed to set on a suitable glass plate and (using an appropriate template/cutter) sample wells and an antiserum trough are prepared. Samples are placed in the wells and the gel plate placed on the bridge of an appropriate electrophoresis chamber (using saturated wicks to maintain contact between gel and buffer solutions). An electric current is applied, sufficient to achieve separation of the constituent proteins. Subsequently, the gel plate is taken out of the electrophoresis chamber and the gel removed from the antiserum trough (it should initially have been cut but not removed). The trough is filled with an appropriate antiserum and diffusion allowed to take place, in a humid chamber overnight. The precipitin lines (arcs) are visualised as described for RID. A polyspecific antiserum may detect a number of proteins in serum, whereas a highly specific antiserum will identify only one type of protein (Figure 10.4).

Immunodeficiency has been used in a broader sense to encompass deficiencies in non-specific immune function. Thus, deficiencies in the complement system, for example, may result in an increased tendency to infection. Specifically, the third component of complement (C3) plays a central role in generating the biologically significant effects of the complement system. These include anaphylactoid and opsonic activity, release of lysosomal enzymes from macrophages and an efflux of leucocytes from the bone marrow. Deficiencies of C3 have been described in animals with persistent, recurrent infections. C3 may be quantified in **fresh** serum (or serum stored at −70°C) using RID. If purified complement components are not available as standards, serum from normal animals can be used to give comparative values.

Other assays of non-specific immunity may test phagocytic/bactericidal function of leucocytes or the ability of specific white cell types to respond to chemotactic stimuli. Such assays are, currently, the exclusive domain of the specialised laboratory and do not lend themselves to 'test kit' methodologies.

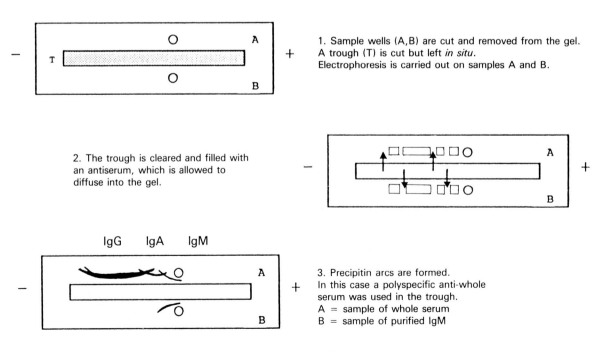

1. Sample wells (A,B) are cut and removed from the gel. A trough (T) is cut but left *in situ*. Electrophoresis is carried out on samples A and B.

2. The trough is cleared and filled with an antiserum, which is allowed to diffuse into the gel.

3. Precipitin arcs are formed. In this case a polyspecific anti-whole serum was used in the trough.
A = sample of whole serum
B = sample of purified IgM

Figure 10.4
Immunoelectrophoresis of Serum Proteins

IMMUNOPROLIFERATIVE DISEASES

In the normal immune response, antibody (=immunoglobulin) producing (lymphoid) cells respond to antigen by controlled division and differentiation. In order to be effective, this cellular response must be under rigid control. Failure in this control system can result in an abnormal proliferation of these cells. The consequence of this proliferation may be twofold.

1. **Lymphoid Tumours.**
    The result of lymphoid neoplasia may be immunosuppression due to interference in the delicate balance between effector cells and suppressor cells within the normal immune response. In some circumstances, lymphoid neoplasia may be associated with autoimmune disease(s) via mechanisms which are not fully understood.

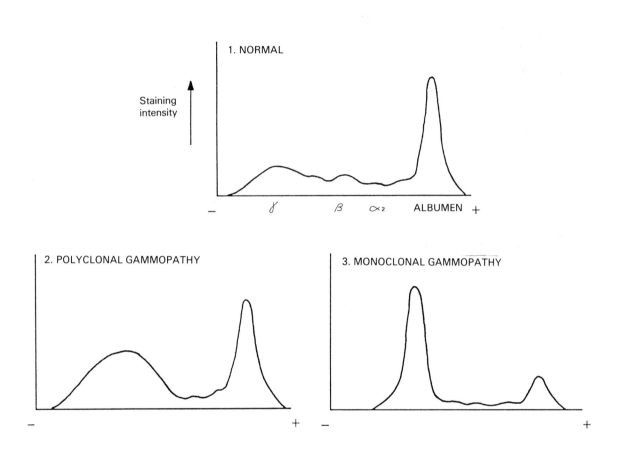

Figure 10.5
Serum Protein Electrophoresis in the Gammopathies

2. **Gammopathies.**
    Malignant transformation of a single antibody-producing lymphoid cell may give rise to the development of a clone of immunoglobulin-producing (tumour) cells. These can usually be distinguished, morphologically, as plasma cells. The plasma cell tumours are known as myelomas or plasmacytomas and because they arise from a single clone, an excess of **homogeneous** immunoglobulin is is produced. This myleoma protein, also termed a paraprotein, is characterised by a rise in a single molecular type of immunoglobulin. This is readily distinguished on an electrophoretic scan as a narrow, sharp peak. This characteristic serum protein pattern is termed

a monoclonal gammopathy and can be diagnosed in the laboratory using simple serum protein electrophoresis. The monoclonal immunoglobulin produced may be of any class (e.g. IgG, IgM, IgA or IgE) and can be specifically characterised using radial immunodiffusion and immuno-electrophoresis. Intact immunoglobulin molecules are composed of heavy chains and light chains. In some monoclonal gammopathies light chains alone are produced or light chains are produced in excess of heavy chains. Since light chains are relatively small they can pass through glomeruli and appear in the urine. These free light chains in urine are termed Bence Jones proteins. They may be detected by electrophoresis (the urine may need to be concentrated). A monoclonal gammopathy characterised by an IgM paraprotein is termed a paraproteinaemia. This condition is frequently associated with hyperviscosity of the blood which has been reported to cause a bleeding disorder, due to impairment of platelet function by the paraprotein.

A polyclonal gammopathy is characterised by an overall rise in gammaglobulin levels, suggesting that multiple cell lines are involved in the production of immunoglobulins. Thus, increases in more than one type of immunoglobulin may be involved and a polyclonal gammopathy is distinguished on serum protein electrophoresis as a broad peak in the globulin region. Figure 10.5 shows the characteristic electrophoretic patterns observed in the gammopathies. A polyclonal gammopathy can occur in a wide variety of pathological conditions e.g. feline infectious peritonitis, Erhlichia canis, rheumatoid arthritis, systemic lupus erythematosus.

ADDITIONAL INFORMATION

FURTHER READING

GORMAN, N.T. and WERNER, L.L. Diagnosis of Immune-mediated Diseases and Interpretation of Immunologic Tests. *Current Veterinary Therapy IX. Small Animal Practice.* W.B. Saunders Company, Philadelphia, PA. (1986). 427-435.

ROSE, N.R., FRIEDMAN, H. and FAHEY, J.L. *Manual of Clinical Laboratory Immunology. (3rd Edition).* American Society for Microbiology, Washington, D.C. (1986).

WEIR, D.M. Application of Immunological Methods in Biomedical Sciences. *Handbook of Experimental Immunology, Volume 3.* Blackwell Scientific Publications. (1986).

For detailed information on fundamental principles of immunology, in an easily readable format, the reader is directed to: —

ROITT, I.M., BROSTOFF, J. and MALE, D.K. *Immunology (1985).* (Churchill Livingstone, Leith Walk, Edinburgh, EH1 3AF) (1985).

CHAPTER 11

POST MORTEM AND BIOPSY EXAMINATIONS

P. J. Brown Ph.D., M.R.C.V.S.

INTRODUCTION

OBJECTIVES OF POST MORTEM AND BIOPSY EXAMINATIONS

An accurate and specific diagnosis is a prerequisite for the proper medical or surgical treatment of a diseased animal and, where appropriate, for the initiation of prophylactic measures in other animals at risk. The increased use of ancillary aids in general practice has allowed the clinician to make accurate and specific diagnoses more frequently but there are certain circumstances where post mortem or biopsy examinations are appropriate and of great value.

Post Mortem Examination

i.   Post mortem examination may be the only method of obtaining a diagnosis in an animal found dead or dying in which no clinical signs have been observed.

ii. It may be necessary to investigate the unexpected death of an animal during or shortly after anaesthesia or operation.

iii. In cases in which no specific diagnosis has been reached, post mortem examination of an animal which has died or on which euthanasia has been performed, may be helpful. Sacrifice of one animal in a group may be the most rapid (and indeed only) way to make a diagnosis and allow appropriate treatment to be commenced among the remainder.

iv. Confirmation of a clinical diagnosis, in an animal which has died or on which euthanasia has been performed, may be requested by the owner. Alternatively, one may wish to correlate clinical and other data with the post mortem findings to understand more fully the pathogenesis of a disease.

Biopsy Examination

i.   Biopsy examination may be used to confirm a diagnosis and, in particular with tumours, to obtain information regarding likely behaviour and hence prognosis.

ii. In other cases, it may clarify a situation in which clinical signs are non-specific or confusing.

Limitations of Post Mortem and Biopsy Examinations

The gross and microscopic appearance of changes in tissue may indicate only the general type of disease process involved. Toxicological or microbiological examination may be needed to provide details. Other diseases, e.g. certain poisons, hypocalcaemia (eclampsia), may produce no pathological lesions.

It takes time for changes that can be seen to occur. In cases of anaesthetic death, for example, depression of CNS function may be so rapid that death occurs before morphological changes can develop.

Some changes, such as pulmonary congestion and oedema or fatty change of the liver, may develop terminally. These should not be taken as evidence of primary disease affecting these tissues. The value of histological examination in particular, is limited by the degree of PM autolysis. This is particularly true with certain tissues or species, e.g. alimentary tract and pancreas, or in neonates, cage birds and laboratory animals which all undergo rapid post mortem change.

The interpretation of the results of histological examination is limited by the selection of a representative sample. A large necrotic tumour may be difficult to diagnose if only a small sample is taken, since the viable tumour tissue may not be included. Inclusion of a portion of normal tissue at the edge of a tumour will often help in assessment of malignancy.

In skin disease, the commonly used punch biopsy yields only a small sample and multiple samples should be obtained. Normal skin has a variable appearance at different sites on the body. Samples from different sites should be identified as such.

COLLECTION AND SELECTION OF SAMPLES

The commonest examination in the laboratory will be of a section of fixed, processed tissue, but other possibilities are impression smears (obtained by gently pressing the cut surface of a lesion against a clean microscope slide) and smears of either abnormal fluid, or washings of the nasal cavity or upper airways, or of cells aspirated from soft tissue masses via a needle and syringe.

Selection of Tissues for Histology

Accurate histological interpretation of lesions requires good preservation of structure. This depends on obtaining samples as soon as possible after death (this is particularly important in the case of certain tissues such as the eye, pancreas, stomach and intestines or nervous tissue). Correct and rapid fixation is also essential (see below).

Select tissues at the edge of a lesion, including a small amount of adjacent normal tissue. This is particularly important in the case of tumours. The presence of invasive growth may be a major indication of malignancy and the centre of a lesion may be necrotic. If there is more than one lesion, or lesions vary in appearance, obtain samples from several sites. They may not all be examined but will be available if required.

Avoid crushing or distortion of the tissues during sampling. This may be a problem in small biopsy specimens removed from poorly accessible sites. Information on histological material requirements in viral diseases is given on page 111, Chapter 9.

Fixation of Tissue

Tissues should be fixed as soon as possible after death or removal from the body. They should be placed in wide-necked (preferably plastic) containers. Use a large volume of fixative in relation to the volume of the tissue to be fixed (about 10 : 1)

The penetration of fixative into a large piece of tissue is slow. Larger portions of friable tissue may be fixed for 24 hours and then cut into smaller pieces. (Brain should be left for at least 96 hours before it is cut up). Peripheral nerve and skeletal muscle will become contracted and distorted if simply immersed in fixative. They should be gently pressed onto cardboard which is then placed in the fixative. Large samples of small intestine are best fixed by tying off both ends of a small loop of bowel and injecting it with fixative before immersion in the normal way. Smaller samples should be pinned on card as above. The most suitable general purpose fixative is formalin (a solution of formaldehyde gas in water). Commercially available solutions are normally 40% formaldehyde (equivalent to 100% formalin). Ten per cent formalin is usually used for fixative, thus requiring a 1 in 10 dilution of the concentrated (40% fomaldehyde) solution. Formalin is poisonous and should be labelled accordingly. Formalin becomes acidic if left for any period of time and this produces unwanted pigment in the tissues. This can be prevented by a few chips of calcium carbonate in the bottom of the container or dilution of the concentrated solution in neutral phosphate buffer rather than water alone.

Other fixatives may be required for specific purposes (e.g. for fixation of eyes or for demonstration of inclusion bodies). Consult the laboratory to which samples are to be sent, for guidance.

METHODS OF EXAMINATION

Equipment required.

The post mortem examination should be considered an essential part of small animal practice. Mention of the small animal practice post mortem room has already been made in the BSAVA publication 'A Manual of Practice Improvement', editor P.B. Fry. Smaller practices may not be able to achieve this ideal but some contamination of premises is inevitable and if suitable facilities are not available, post mortem examinations are likely to be infrequent and incomplete and therefore unsatisfactory.

To facilitate cleaning, equipment to be used in the post mortem room should be kept to a minimum and instruments and protective clothing reserved excusively for use there.

Instruments required are as follows:

Scissors (large and fine)
Rat-toothed forceps
Bone forceps (large and fine)
Stainless steel saw (or Desoutter cast cutter)
Large knife
Small scalpel
A cork board and dissection darts are useful for pinning out the carcass of rodents, cage birds and neonatal animals.

Protective clothing should include rubber gloves, rubber boots, protective boiler suit and a plastic or rubber apron. On some occasions a face mask and head cover are needed.

POST MORTEM EXAMINATION PROCEDURES IN CATS AND DOGS.

The aim of a post mortem examination is a thorough investigation of all organs and tissues of the different body systems. To facilitate this, a standard sequence of examination should be adopted and all organs should be examined, even when clinical history does not indicate disease affecting them. Clinically significant lesions may be missed in hurried and incomplete examinations, while a careful and complete examination frequently reveals unexpected but significant information.

Before starting, you should consider all the information available, including the clinical findings, radiographic evidence and laboratory results.

The following is a suitable brief guide to post mortem examination. In exceptional circumstances you may need to modify the standard procedure.

1. **Note age, sex, breed, weight.**

2. **External inspection.**

Assess the general state of bodily condition and examine the anus, genitalia, limbs, skin and mucous membranes of mouth, nose, eyes and ears.

There may be soiling of skin associated with discharge from the eyes, ears, mouth, nose, anus, vulva or penis. Pale mucous membranes may indicate shock or anaemia. Jaundice may be seen as yellowing of the mucous membranes and sclera and reddening or haemorrhages of mucous membranes may be present associated with septicaemia or viraemia. Sunken eyes and dehydrated skin may be due to loss of body fluid or may be seen in death from shock. Tumours of the skin, subcutaneous tissue or mammary glands may be visible or palpable; in some cases even small skin tumours may have resulted in widespread metastasis to other, distant sites. Skin wounds or torn claws may be present in cases of road traffic accidents.

Brief immersion in water, of animals of long coated breeds, will reduce spread of hair to viscera during the examination which follows.

Abnormalities should be recorded as accurately as possible as they are found. Description of the lesions should include number, location, size, shape, colour and consistency. Samples for histological or microbiological examination should be taken from each lesion as it is encountered. They may not be subsequently submitted for further examination but they will often be difficult to relocate at the end of a complete examination.

Interpretation of the findings should wait until the post mortem has been completed and, where appropriate, the results of histological or microbiological examinations are known.

3. Reflect the limbs.

Lay the animal on its back. Cut the skin and muscle in the axilla and inguinal regions on each side. The hip joints should be incised and examined. The limbs will then lie flat, away from the body which will remain upright and stable.

4. Midline skin incision.

Incise the skin in midline from the mandibular symphysis to the pelvis; in a male dog the incision should be taken to one side of the penis. The skin should be reflected over the ventral and lateral aspects of the carcase. There may be signs of dehydration, haemorrhage or oedema. The occurrence of subcutaneous oedema may be associated with accumulation of fluid elsewhere in the carcase.

5. Reflect the tongue.

6. Examine superficial lymph nodes.

The following nodes should be examined: popliteal (lying caudal to the stifle joint), superficial inguinal (embedded in subcutaneous fat cranial to the pelvis), prescapular (cranial to the scapula) and submandibular (ventral to the angle of the jaw, cranial to the submandibular salivary glands — often more than one lymph node present). Lesions may be present in a lymph node which is not obviously enlarged. Lymph nodes should be incised and their cut surfaces examined for normal differentiation into cortex and medulla, and the presence of focal lesions.

7. Expose trachea.

Remove the muscles from the ventral aspect of the trachea. Cut through the muscles attached to the medial borders of the horizontal rami of the mandibles and pull the tongue out ventrally. Cut through the articulations of the hyoid bones and strip the oesophagus and trachea down to the thoracic inlet.

8. Lymph nodes/Tonsil.

Examine the retropharyngeal lymph nodes. These nodes are located caudal to the submandibular salivary glands and dorsal to the larynx and tonsils. Both may be enlarged in lymphosarcoma. Enlarged tonsils protrude from the crypts. Enlargement and reddening of the tonsils indicates inflammation. Irregular enlargement of one tonsil by firm, white tissue is seen with spread of squamous carcinoma of the epithelium of the tonsillar crypt; there may be extension to local lymph nodes.

9. Reflect the skin and open the abdominal cavity.

Make a small incision through the linea alba and check for the presence of free fluid in the abdominal cavity, which may then be collected and sampled. Open the abdomen from the xiphisternum to the pubic symphysis and reflect the abdominal wall laterally.

Inspect the abdominal viscera in situ. Note the type and volume of any exudate, the appearance of the parietal and visceral peritoneum, the relationships of the major organs and the presence of any major vascular anomalies.

A few millilitres of clear, colourless fluid is normally present and normal peritoneal surfaces are smooth and glistening.

10. Open the thorax by removing the sternum.

Make a small incision in the diaphragm and note the inrush of air (indicating a normal negative pressure in the pleural cavity). If pneumothorax is suspected the incision into the diaphragm should be made with the chest submerged in water and the formation of any gas bubbles noted. Note the amount and type of any abnormal pleural fluid.

Separate the diaphragm from the last rib to allow insertion of rib cutters. Clear a cutting line through the soft tissues of the right thoracic wall. Cut through the ribs with rib cutters so that about two-thirds of the ventral rib cage is removed. Reflect the rib cage over to the left hand side, cutting through the sternal attachments of the mediastinum, and break or cut through the ribs to expose the thoracic viscera in situ, noting, in particular, the appearance of pleural surfaces, the presence of any thymus or thymic tumour, the lungs, heart and major blood vessels.

Clear the connective tissue attachments around the trachea and oesophagus at the thoracic inlet and apply traction to separate the thoracic viscera from the dorsal aspect of the thorax.

11. Locate and examine the adrenal glands.

The left adrenal gland lies cranial and slightly medial to the left kidney. The right gland lies nearer the hilus of the right kidney. Incise both glands longitudinally. The pale cortex should conform roughly to the shape of the gland. The central medulla is softer and red/brown in colour. The cortex and medulla should be present in about equal proportions.

12. Structural relationships.

Examine structure and relationship of major structures and organs of the oral cavity, pharynx, thorax and abdomen.

13. Removal of organs.

Remove tongue and thoracic organs together, with or without abdominal organs. Leave the urogenital tract in the abdomen.

Applying traction caudally, incise the dorsolateral margins of the diaphragm. Cut the mesentery close to its dorsal attachments allowing the thoracic organs attached to the stomach, intestines and liver, together with the omentum, spleen and mesentery, to be withdrawn. The rectum may be transected cranial to the pelvis or, if appropriate, the bones of the pelvic floor should be removed. The kidneys and ureters (and ovaries and uterus in entire female animals) are left in situ.

14. Examination of the alimentary system.

Upper alimentary tract.

Inspect the teeth, gums, oropharyngeal mucosa and salivary glands. Examine the tongue and oesophagus. Incise the latter along its length and study the mucosal surface.

Gastrointestinal tract.

Examine the structure and relationships of the excised organs. Cut the omentum and mesentery along their serosal margins and examine the mesenteric lymph nodes. Incise the stomach (along the greater curvature) and intestines along their entire length and examine serosal and mucosal surfaces. Apply gentle pressure to the gall bladder — bile will enter the duodenum from the common bile duct, if the latter is patent. Remove the oesophagus, stomach and intestines from the other viscera.

15. Pancreas.

Examine for size, shape and colour.

16. Liver.

Examine the surface of the liver and the gall bladder. Make several cuts into all-lobes and incise the gall bladder. Cystic hyperplasia of the gall bladder mucosa is a common incidental senile change in dogs. The gall bladder may be distended in animals which have not eaten recently. Enlargement of the liver occurs in various diseases and is usually associated with rounding of the edges of the lobes.

17. Spleen.

Remove the spleen from its omental attachments and incise. The spleen may be diffusely or irregularly enlarged. The normal structure is composed of red and white pulp.

18. Examine the thyroid and parathyroid glands.

The thyroid gland on each side lies caudal to the larynx on the lateral aspect of the trachea. Usually, 2 small, pale parathyroid glands are present, one close to and one embedded in each thyroid gland.

19. Respiratory tract.

Examine the larynx, trachea and mediastinum. Palpate and inspect both lungs. Open the larynx and cut down the trachea and major bronchi; examine the cut surfaces of the lungs.

20. Heart and Pericardium.

Examine the pericardial sac. Cut through the pericardium and expose the heart.

Examine the heart for enlargement or abnormality of shape. Enlargement of the right side makes the heart bigger and rounded. An enlargement of the left side makes the heart bigger and longer. The muscle wall of the right ventricle is normally much thinner than the left. Enlargement may be a result of dilation of the chamber and/or hypertrophy of the muscle wall. Both are normal compensatory mechanisms to increase cardiac output and occur in highly trained animals, e.g. greyhounds, as well as in animals with chronic cardiac disease. The significance and interpretation of such changes is determined by clinical history and other PM findings.

Examine the chambers of the heart in detail. Hold the heart with the anterior surface uppermost. The longitudinal groove (corresponding to the interventricular septum) runs diagonally from lower left to upper right of the heart. The left ventricle and atrium lie to the right of the groove, the right ventricle and atrium to the left.

Cut into the auricular appendage and lateral wall of the right atrium and expose the right AV valve. Examine the atrium and valve. Cut through the valve and the wall of the right ventricle, along its cranial border, to the apex of the heart. Examine the chordae tendinae and the valvular and mural endocardium. Cut through the pulmonary valve to expose the lumenal surface of the pulmonary trunk.

Incise and examine the left atrium, left ventricle and aorta in a similar way.

21. Examination of blood vessels.

The position and size of vessels should be studied and the lumenal surfaces examined.

22. Urinary system.

Examine the kidneys, ureters, bladder (and prostate in the male dog) in situ. Apply gentle pressure to the bladder and check for patency of the urethra. The entire urinary tract may be removed for dissection, or each part excised and examined separately. Incise the kidneys longitudinally and strip off the capsule carefully. The kidneys of the dog and cat differ markedly in shape and colour. The kidney of the cat is pale and surface blood vessels are prominent; the capsule strips very readily. The kidney of the dog is bean shaped and dark red; the capsule may be removed easily but occasional fine fibrous strands penetrate the cortical tissue. Inspect the capsular surface and the cut surface and check that the cortex and medulla are present in a uniform , correct proportion. In neonatal animals the cortex is normally very thin. Examine the renal pelvis.

23. Ureters/Bladder.

The ureters may be distended by urine or pus in association with hydronephrosis or pyelonephritis. Anomalous development of the ureters may occur. The most commonly recognised problem is ectopic ureter in the bitch where a ureter opens into the urethra or genital tract distal to the trigone of the bladder, resulting in incontinence.

Examine the serosal and mucosal surfaces of the incised bladder.

24. Male genital system.

A small amount of discharge from the preputial orifice is normal in dogs. The prostate may have to be examined at the same time as the bladder and urethra. Differentiation between hyperplasia, infection and neoplasia depends particularly on size, shape and structure. In castrated dogs the prostate is small. Palpate the testes within the scrotum which should also be examined. Incise the scrotum and expose the testes. Section each testis and epididymis. Normal testicular tissue is fawn coloured, fleshy and bulges on cutting.

25. Female genital system.

Examine the ovaries and uterus in situ. Unless contraindicated they can be removed by cutting at the cervix, and the vagina may not be examined routinely.

26. Musculoskeletal system — joints, bones, muscle.

Joints: The hip joints are incised at an early stage in PM examination. They are the site of specific diseases which are well recognised in different ages and breeds of dogs. Other synovial joints are examined when indicated. Note the amount and character of synovial fluid, the appearance of synovial membranes and the conformation and appearance of articular surfaces.

Examination of the intervertebral disc joints requires opening of the spinal canal. This procedure will be described later.

Bones: Softness of ribs may be noted when they are cut to expose the thoracic organs. Other bones are examined as required. Use bone forceps to open the shaft of the femur and expose the bone marrow. In adult animals the marrow is pale pink, fatty and floats in fixative. Leukaemia is associated with infiltration and replacement of the marrow by tumour cells. The hypercellular marrow is more solid, red/pink in colour and sinks in fixative.

Muscle: The craniomandibular muscles particularly, are affected in atrophic myositis and eosinophilic myositis. In the latter case they may be swollen, but histological confirmation may be required. Atrophy of muscle will occur in any wasting disease and develops locally if nerve supply is damaged.

27. Nervous system.

The brachial plexus is exposed early on when the axilla is incised. Other nerves may be examined if indicated. Examination of the brain and spinal cord should not be neglected if disease affecting those parts is suspected. With practice, the time taken to expose the central nervous system is not great. In many cases, a grossly evident lesion, e.g. hydrocephalus, a disc protrusion or a tumour mass will be readily seen. In other cases, e.g encephalitis, no macroscopic lesion may be apparent but marked histological lesions are present. Other cases will occur in which no lesion is detected even after microscopic examination.

The brain and spinal cord may be exposed together or the head may be removed by disarticulation of the atlanto-occipital joint. Reflect the skin and muscle from the dorsal spinous process of the vertebrae and then cut through and remove the dorsal parts of the vertebral arches to expose the spinal cord. Using bone forceps or a saw, cut through the sinus of the frontal bone into the anterior border of the cranial cavity. Continue the incision on each side along the lateral aspects of the skull to the foramen magnum. Prise up the roof of the cranium and remove it. Ensure that the leaf-like projections of the parietal bone between the cerebrum and cerebellum are removed. Incise the spinal cord caudal to the foramen magnum.

Spinal cord: Ideally the spinal cord, or the portion of it containing a potential lesion, should be fixed in situ for 12—24 hours. It may then be more easily removed, without damaging it. Remove the spinal cord by grasping the dura at one end and lift gently to expose the spinal nerves which are then cut. Avoid pulling the cord. Examine the dura and cord for areas of compression, haemorrhage, necrosis or tumour growth. Examine the ventral surface of the spinal canal for evidence of protrusion of intervertebral discs and cut through and examine one or more discs for evidence of degenerative change.

Brain: Remove the dura if it remains attached. The brain may be fixed in situ or after removal. Unless samples for microbiology etc. are required, examination of the fixed brain is easier and more rewarding. Turn the head upside down and cut through cranial nerves and olfactory bulbs and allow the brain to fall gently out of the cavity. Examine the floor of the cranium, the pituitary gland and pituitary fossa.

External inspection of the brain (preferably after fixation) will frequently reveal no specific changes. However, tumours or cerebellar hypoplasia, for example, may be visible. Swelling of the brain may cause protrusion of the caudal cerebellum through the foramen magnum. This is evident as a cone shaped compression.

Examination of internal structure of the brain is best delayed until it has been fixed for at least 96 hours. Section the brain transversely at regular 0.5 — 1.0 cm intervals. Examine the ventricles and the white and grey matter.

28. **Ears, eyes and nasal cavity.**

Ears: Open the vertical canal and examine the external ear canal. Carefully remove the tympanic bulla with bone forceps to expose the middle ear.

Eyes: Grasp the closed eyelids with forceps and incise the lid margins. Apply gentle traction and cut through the soft tissues surrounding the globe and section the optic nerve. Any soft tissue attached to the eye should be removed before it is fixed.

Nasal cavity: Divide the skull longitudinally along the midline and examine the nasal cavities. The frontal sinuses are also exposed.

POST MORTEM TECHNIQUE IN LABORATORY ANIMALS

Post mortem autolysis develops rapidly in laboratory animals and examination should not be delayed.

The technique is essentially that just described. It is helpful to immobilise the carcase on its back, with limbs abducted, by the use of adhesive tapes or pins and a cork board.

POST MORTEM TECHNIQUE IN CAGE BIRDS

The risk of psittacosis should always be remembered when examining birds. A surgical cap and mask should be worn and the bird should be soaked in a 2% lysol solution to prevent spread of infection by dust aerosol. Equipment (instruments, cork boards, pins, trays etc) should be disinfected after use. The diagnosis of psittacosis is mentioned elsewhere in this manual (see page 93).

1. Soak the carcase and pin the bird out, on its back, on a cork board.

2. Incise and reflect the skin and feathers from the ventral neck, thorax and abdomen.

3. Incise the muscle of the ventral abdominal wall and extend the incision cranially through the pectoral muscles, ribs, coracoid and clavicle to remove the sternum and pectoral muscles. This exposes the thoracic and abdominal viscera and air sacs. Examine the different body systems. The position of most of the organs is straight forward. The range of changes which can occur in them resembles those in mammals but there are certain anatomical differences:-

Respiratory system

This includes the nasal cavity and sinuses, oropharynx, the trachea, lungs and air sacs. Lesions of the air sacs include accumulation of exudate within them and thickening or cloudiness of their serous linings. The lungs of birds are normally adherent to the ribs and blunt dissection is required to remove them.

Alimentary system

The different regions to examine are the coelomic cavities, the oropharynx, oesophagus (and crop), stomach, (glandular portion and gizzard), small intestine, large intestine (including paired caeca) and cloaca. The pancreas lies in the mesentery of the duodenal loop. The liver consists of left and right major lobes. In small birds, it is normally necessary to remove all the organs together. If microbiological examination is not required, brief fixation will aid subsequent investigation of different regions.

Urogenital system

The kidneys are paired elongated organs with obvious lobulations. In females, the reproductive structure on the left side only are functional. The ovary may be greatly enlarged by developing follicles at times of sexual activity. Regions of the left oviduct are the infundibulum, magnum, isthmus, uterus and vagina. In males, the testes are bean-shaped and located near the cranial end of the kidney. The left testis is usually larger than the right and the size of both increases with sexual activity.

Lymphoreticular system

The spleen is a small rounded structure in the mesentery of the glandular stomach (proventriculus). True lymph nodes occur only in aquatic birds. In other species, solitary lymphoid nodules are scattered through the parenchymatous organs.

DESCRIPTION AND INTERPRETATION OF COMMON LESIONS

Lymph Nodes

Lymphosarcoma: Affected lymph nodes are often greatly enlarged and composed of soft, pale cream tissue. Usually, several lymph nodes will be affected. There may be no distinction between cortex and medulla in advanced cases. Early cases may require histological examination.

Reactive hyperplasia: During reaction to local or systemic infection, proliferation of lymphoid cells in lymph nodes may cause enlargement of lymph nodes in which lymphoid follicles are visible in the cortex.

Lymphadenitis: Oedema, congestion, haemorrhage or abscess formation may occur in a node draining a focus of infection.

Tumour metastases: A lymph node may be largely replaced by secondary deposits of a tumour. The tumour tissue will resemble that at the primary site and remnants of normal lymphoid tissue will usually be visible at the periphery.

Abdominal and Thoracic Cavity

Ascitic fluid: This is watery, straw coloured or may be blood tinged; peritoneal surfaces are smooth and shiny.

Exudate from a peritonitis: This is more viscid, cloudy and may contain fibrin clots; the peritoneum has a dull, finely granular, often congested surface and there may be deposits of fibrin. In some cases of Feline Infectious Peritonitis, this may be an obvious clinical or post mortem finding. In other, non-effusive cases, however, little or no fluid is produced.

If there is heamoperitoneum the presence of blood clots around a damaged vessel may reveal the site of haemorrhage: you are unlikely to locate the site of haemorrhage once the organs have been removed.

Obstruction of the hepatic portal vein within the liver may lead to the development of an accessory portal circulation. A prominent plexus of vessels draining into the renal vein may be obvious. Other channels are the intercostal, gastric and oesophageal veins to the azygos vein.

In addition to the types of fluid described in the abdominal cavity, damage to the thoracic duct lymphatic vessel may lead to chylothorax. The fluid is cloudy white or pink and characterised by the presence of fat. The site of damage is very difficult to locate.

Adrenal Glands

Nodular hyperplasia: Multiple nodular lesions of tissue resembling normal cortex extend into the medulla or into the capsule around the gland. These lesions are common in old dogs. In many cases they are incidental findings but may be associated with hyperadrenocorticism resulting in Cushing's Disease. The adrenal lesions may be secondary to a lesion in the pituitary or hypothalmus resulting in excess production of adrenocorticotrophic hormone. Some pituitary adenomas will only be visible histologically.

Calcification: This is a not uncommon incidental finding in old animals.

Tumours of the cortex or medulla are less common conditions. These may be locally invasive, typically infiltrating the vena cava, and may metastasize.

Upper Alimentary Tract

Pigmentation of the buccal mucosa may be present and may extend into the oesophagus.

Nodular gingival hyperplasia (epulis): This is a common incidental finding in older dogs. Other gingival tumours include fibrosarcomas, squamous cell carcinomas and melanomas which are malignant and may be locally infiltrative or metastasize.

Ulceration of the oral or lingual epithelium may be associated with dental problems or may occur in uraemia.

Salivary gland tumours are uncommon. They are usually malignant.

Gastrointestinal Tract

Haemorrhagic erosions and ulcers of the gastric mucosa, together with oral and lingual ulceration, frequently accompany uraemia. Shallow stress ulcers may also occur in a range of other disease states.

Hyperaemia of the stomach and intestine is normally associated with feeding, and reddening of the intestine develops rapidly as a PM change. Where histological examination is required for confirmation, samples should be obtained very soon after death. A suitable method is described under Selection of Tissues for Histology (see page 130).

Gastritis and enteritis produce reddening of the mucosa and sometimes of the serosal surface. The intestinal contents are often abnormally fluid and there may be a haemorrhagic or mucoid exudate or sloughing of necrotic epithelium (diphtheresis).

Thickening of the intestinal wall may occur associated with chronic inflammation or neoplasia. In chronic enteritis the intestine is not congested but there is diffuse thickening due to cellular infiltration of the mucosa and/or hypertrophy of the muscle wall.

Lymphosarcoma may produce a similar appearance but often the lesions are more localised and larger and mesenteric lymph nodes are frequently enlarged due to replacement by tumour cells..

In cases of carcinoma, the mucosa is usually ulcerated and the wall of the stomach or intestines is markedly thickened by firm white tissue. The lumen of the intestine may be narrowed or obstructed. There may be obvious serosal extension and nodules of firm white tissue may be present in local lymph nodes. **Smooth muscle tumours** may be large but are usually benign.

Pancreas

This gland contains both exocrine and endocrine tissue.

Patchy, dark red discolouration of the pancreas is a common incidental, agonal change. The following diseases of exocrine tissue produce fairly characteristic lesions.

Endocrine insufficiency: In young dogs, degeneration or failure of development of exocrine tissue results in the pancreas being thin and lace-like. In older dogs, inflammation and scarring may produce a small, irregular, fibrotic pancreas in which exocrine tissue is reduced. In both cases (pancreatic atrophy or hypoplasia and chronic pancreatitis) deficiency of enzymes results in poor digestion of food leading to weight loss and the passage of pale, bulky faeces.

Acute haemorrhagic pancreatic necrosis (necrotising pancreatitis): This lesion, due to the lytic effects of the exocrine enzymes, results in multiple focal lesions in the pancreas and surrounding fat. There may be haemorrhage and necrosis in the pancreas and necrosis of fat resulting in small, chalky white lesions.

Nodular hyperplasia: Single or multiple raised nodules of slightly pale tissue are a common, incidental finding in old dogs. Larger lesions may be indistinguishable from benign tumours.

Interstitial pancreatitis with patchy inflammation and fibrosis, causing a finely granular surface, is not usually associated with clinical disease.

Pancreatic carcinoma: Malignant exocrine tumours typically arise at the head of the pancreas. At this site, the large, hard, white tumour may obstruct the bile duct. There may be a spread of tumour to the liver and local lymph nodes.

Lesions of islet cells — include hyperplasia and neoplasia: In each case, a small, single, nodular lesion may present. Differentiation from nodular hyperplasia of exocrine tissue and assessment of malignancy, require histological examination. The clinical significance will depend on the amount and type (determined by the cells involved) of hormone produced. Even small primary or secondary deposits of tumour tissue may have marked clinical effects.

Diabetes mellitus: This is the commonest pancreatic endocrine disease seen in the dog and cat. The diagnosis is largely made on clinical and biochemical grounds. Gross lesions in the pancreas are often absent or incidental and histological examination frequently fails to reveal a lesion. PM changes occur rapidly and tissue should be fixed as soon as possible after death. The most obvious PM lesion in cases of diabetes mellitus is fatty change of the liver.

The Liver

Gallstones (Choleliths): These are rare and usually asymptomatic.

Inflammation: In infectious canine hepatitis, the liver may be enlarged and has a mottled appearance due to focal necrosis. There may be fibrin strands and petechial haemorrhage on the capsule. The wall of the gall bladder is often thickened due to oedema. In some other diseases, the liver may be enlarged but show only vague mottling or an exaggerated lobular pattern. Microscopic examination may reveal obvious lesions.

Fatty change: The liver is enlarged, pale and obviously fatty. This degenerative change occurs in various toxic, infectious or metabolic diseases and in starvation. It is the major, gross lesion present in cases of diabetes mellitus.

Chronic venous congestion: In congestive cardiac failure, the liver is enlarged and the lobular architecture is exagerated due to a combination of venous congestion and fatty change of liver cells. This results in the mottled red/pale yellow appearance of the so called 'nutmeg liver'. In later stages, fibrosis may occur, causing a reduction in size and increased firmness on cutting.

Hyperplasia: Pale, rounded nodules of tissue of fairly normal consistency are sometimes seen in old animals in which they are incidental findings. They may also be seen in cases of cirrhosis.

Cirrhosis: The liver is small, firm and irregular in shape due to intermingled areas of fibrosis and nodular hyperplasia. Accessory portal veins may be present, secondary to vascular obstruction in the liver.

Neoplasia: The liver may be a site of tumour metastasis and primary tumours of the liver may arise from the hepatocytes or the epithelial cells of the bile ducts. The hepatocellular tumours may form large, single or multiple masses of tissue which may be pale and soft. Malignant tumours may spread locally but can remain within a single lobe of the liver and histological examination is needed to distinguish them from a grossly similar benign lesion. Bile duct carcinomas generally result in multiple nodules of firm, white tissue and resemble secondary deposits of carcinoma from other sites.

Lymphosarcoma: This may produce nodular lesions in the liver or there may be more diffuse infiltration. Diffuse infiltration may also occur in cases of lymphoid or myeloid leukaemia in which diseases other tissues such as bone marrow, lymph nodes and the spleen, will also be affected.

Congenital portosystemic shunts: These are usually associated with a small liver. The shunting vessel may be intrahepatic or extrahepatic. In some cases, no abnormal vessel is seen but histological examination may reveal an abnormality of the intrahepatic vasculature.

The Spleen

Congestion: This is common in many conditions, e.g. congestive cardiac failure, toxaemias, barbiturate poisoning and may occur in cases of gastric torsion. An identical gross appearance is seen in haemolytic anaemia.

Nodular hyperplasia: This is a common lesion in old dogs and appears as one or more nodules, usually up to about 3cm in diameter, protruding from the capsule. The cut surface is pale with intermingled red areas. Some nodules are larger and there may be haemorrhage from them. The macroscopic appearance is similar to that of some splenic tumours, from which they need to be distinguished.

Haemangioma/Haemangiosarcoma: These tumours may have a similar macroscopic appearance, producing large, rounded masses of soft, red tissue. In both cases there may be haemorrhage. The benign tumour is composed largely of clotted blood. The malignant tumour has more solid tissue areas and metastases are often present elsewhere. In the absence of metastasis, histological examination is required to distinguish haemangioma from haemangiosarcoma.

Lymphosarcoma/Leukaemia: In these diseases there may be diffuse infiltration by tumour cells. In lymphosarcoma, the nodules of white pulp may be enlarged or there may be more solid tumour masses. In leukaemia, the red pulp is increased in extent and composed of soft pale red tissue.

Siderofibrotic plaques: These lesions are of little significance. They appear as crusty grey/green thickened areas, confined to the capsule.

Thyroid and Parathyroid Glands

Thyroid adenitis — inflammation of the thyroid is likely to result in enlargement and usually will be associated with obvious inflammation in adjacent tissues.

Thyroid atrophy: Gross reduction in size of the thyroid will be associated with reduced production of thyroid hormones and may be seen in clinical hypothyroidism.

Thyroid hyperplasia: Enlargement may occur as a physiological response to increased demand. Deficiency of iodine, which would result in a compensatory hyperplasia, is unlikely to occur in normal diets for small animals. Clinical hyperthyroidism is rare in dogs but is not uncommon in older cats. Both glands will be enlarged and composed of fairly normal tissue.

Thyroid neoplasia: Benign or malignant tumours may produce a large mass which may be unilateral or involve both glands. With some carcinomas there may be obvious local invasion or metastasis but with others, microscopic examination may be needed to distinguish them from adenomas. Some 'heart base' tumours arise from ectopic thyroid tissue.

Parathyroid hyperplasia: Uniform enlargement of all glands is usually secondary, due to hyperphosphataemia as a result of chronic renal disease or nutritional imbalance of calcium and phosphate. In either case, increased secretion of parathyroid hormone leads to resorption of mineral from bone and this may lead to 'rubber jaw'. Primary hyperplasia and benign or malignant tumours are rare.

The Respiratory Tract

Reduction of the lumen of the airways may be caused by deformity, inflammatory or tumour nodules, or exudate. The nature of the latter will vary, depending on the precise cause and may be associated with similar exudate in the bronchial tree.

Mediastinum: A feature which may be seen in the bronchial and mediastinal lymph nodes is the presence of black pigment in otherwise normal nodes. Similar pigment may be present in the lungs and merely indicates that the animal has lived in an urban environment. Anterior mediastinal masses of solid white tissue include thymomas and thymic lymphosarcomas.

Lung: The pleura may be dull, thickened or roughened due to pleurisy. There may be adhesions between visceral and parietal pleura and an excess of pleural fluid. There may be pneumonia in the underlying lung tissue. Normal lung tissue is pink, spongy and floats in water or formalin. The lung lobes will normally have deflated slightly when the thorax was opened. All or part of the lung may be affected by lesions resulting in changes in the size, colour and consistency of the lungs.

Anthracosis: Minute spots and flecks of black pigment in the lungs and local lymph nodes merely indicates life in an urban environment.

Congestion: The congested lung is slightly swollen and dark red, but is still spongy and floats. Blood exudes from the surface. Congestion may occur terminally and hypostatic congestion may develop in a dependent lung or lobes. In congestive cardiac failure there is frequently pulmonary congestion and oedema.

Oedema: Frothy oedema fluid is present in the trachea and bronchial tree and exudes or can be readily expressed from the cut surface. The colour is normal or slightly pale but oedema and congestion may occur together in heart failure.

Bronchopneumonia: In acute lesions, the affected lung is dark red and exudation of fluid and cells, together with a reduction in the amount of air in the bronchioles and alveoli, results in consolidation of the lung parenchyma, which sinks in water or formalin. Mucopurulent fluid exudes from bronchioles on cut surface. The overlying pleura may be involved.

In chronic lesions, affected lung is grey/brown in colour, collapsed below the level of surrounding normal lung, and firm due to fibrosis. Most cases of bronchopneumonia are caused by inhalation of airborne pathogens and lead to lesions in the central and ventral parts of the lungs. In embolic pneumonia (due to haematogenous spread) multiple, smaller lesions are scattered throughout all lobes; they may form obvious lung abscesses. Aspiration pneumonia, resulting from inhalation of food, vomitus or other material, results in a severe, acute necrotising lesion in the cranioventral parts.

Emphysema: The accumulation of air in enlarged respiratory bronchioles or air spaces, appears as small gas bubbles. They may be visible beneath the pleura and on cut surfaces and there may be crepitation on palpation. Affected portions of lung are pale pink/grey, may be swollen and bear imprints of the ribs. Emphysema may occur in chronic bronchopneumonia as a result of coughing and inflammation of the bronchiolar walls. In some cases air may escape from the lungs and enter mediastinal tissue; this may also occur due to trauma.

Collapse: The collapse of a lung will occur in pneumothorax or hydrothorax. The affected lung tissue is obviously shrunken and the pleura may appear diffusely thickened. The poorly inflated lungs appear dark red in colour and float poorly.

Heart and Pericardium

Hydropericardium: The pericardial sac contains an excess of clear serous fluid. Similar fluid may be present subcutaneously and in other body cavities. The pericardium and epicardium are smooth and shiny.

Pericarditis: Pericardial and epicardial surfaces are thickened and dull, and there may be fibrin deposition and fibrin clots in the pericardial fluid.

Congenital lesions: These will often be seen in young animals and may be single or multiple. They include ventricular and atrial septal defects, valvular defects causing incompetence and allowing reflux of blood, and narrowing or stenosis of valves restricting blood flow; there may often be a post-stenotic dilation.

There may also be anomalous development of major blood vessels which is discussed below.

Bacterial endocarditis: Bacterial infection of the heart valves leads to valvular endocarditis; the valves are irregularly thickened by friable red/white tissue. Embolism may lead to thrombosis and infarction elsewhere. The left AV valve of dogs is most commonly affected.

Endocardiosis: This is a degenerative change which increases with advancing age and is a common lesion in old dogs. The left AV valve is the most common site. The valve, and sometimes the chordae tendinae, are thickened or distorted by firm, pale tissue. The endocardial surface is smooth and shiny. Mild lesions are of little significance.

Uraemic endocardial degeneration: In cases of chronic renal failure with uraemia, degenerative changes in subendocardial tissue may occur. This may lead to white fibrous, sometimes calcified, plaques in the left atrium or elsewhere, often termed mural endocarditis. There may sometimes be thrombosis.

Myocarditis: Bacterial myocarditis may occur as part of a generalised infection. Parvovirus infection of the myocardium in very young dogs may lead to acute or chronic heart failure; the more common manifestation of infection is that of gastroenteritis in weaned and adult animals.

Cardiomyopathy: Primary disease of the heart muscle may occur in dogs (particularly large and giant breeds) and in cats. In dogs and cats an enlarged dilated heart is the only consistent feature. In cats, thrombosis of the endocardium or the aorta may also be found.

Blood Vessels

Congenital anomalies: These may occur — common ones include patent ductus arteriosus and right sided aortic arch. The latter defect is important because of the obstruction of the oesophagus produced by the vascular ring. Congenital porto systemic shunts are another example of a vascular abnormality in which clinical signs are not primarily related to the cardiovascular system.

Thrombosis: Thrombotic material is firmly adherent to the vessel wall and may occur as a result of embolism due to bacterial endocarditis. In cats, thrombosis in the distal aorta or femoral arteries may occur in association with cardiomyopathy. Extensive thrombosis in pulmonary blood vessels may occur in cases of renal amyloidosis or Cushing's disease in dogs.

Arteriosclerotic changes: These appear as plaques near the origins of major arterial branches, and may occur in the abdominal aorta of dogs. Such lesions do not have the significance they do in man.

The Urinary Tract

Infarction: A recent infarct is wedge shaped, extending from the corticomedullary junction to the cortical surface, and is red or pale with a red margin. Healing leads to focal firm, white, depressed cortical scars.

Acute interstitial nephritis: This is rarely seen in cats but is sometimes seen in leptospirosis in dogs. The kidney is enlarged and the cut surface bulges. There may be hyperaemia of vessels at the corticomedullary junction and pale spots or streaks in the cortex caused by cellular infiltration. Some cases of acute interstitial nephritis may recover, but develop eventually into a chronic interstitial nephritis. The appearance in such cases, due to extensive and progressive fibrosis, is that of an end-stage kidney.

End-stage kidney: The kidneys are small and pale and the capsular surface is irregular, pitted or finely granular.

The kidney is firm to cut and the capsule may be adherent to areas of scar tissue. The cortex, particularly, is reduced in thickness and often irregular, and bands of fibrous tissue extend into the kidney from the capsular surface. Multiple small cysts may be present in scarred areas, particularly at the corticomedullary junction. Occasional small streaks of fibrous scarring are a common incidental finding in old cats and dogs.

A kidney of this type represents the end-stage of a chronic process and may be due to chronic interstitial nephritis (due to infection with leptospira or some other organism), chronic glomerulonephritis, chronic nephrotoxicity, renal dysplasia or even chronic pyelonephritis. These different causes may be impossible to distinguish, even histologically.

Glomerulonephritis: In acute glomerulonephritis, the kidneys are slightly enlarged. The cortex appears swollen and may be rather pale. The glomeruli may appear as minute pale or red spots. Chronic glomerulonephritis may develop in less severe cases in which progressive fibrosis leads to the development of an end-stage kidney.

Amyloidosis: In renal amyloidosis the kidneys are enlarged and pale. The cortex appears swollen and pale. Glomeruli are prominent on close inspection. In cats, medullary deposition may occur with necrosis of the renal papillae and signs of acute renal failure.

Hydronephrosis: Retention of urine within the renal pelvis leads to progressive dilation of the pelvis with loss of medullary, and eventually cortical, tissue. The lesion is due to chronic urinary obstruction. Depending on the site, hydroureter may also occur.

Pyelonephritis: This refers to infection within both the renal pelvis and parenchyma. The renal pelvis may become distended by purulent fluid (pyonephrosis) and in the parenchyma foci of necrosis and fibrous scar tissue may coexist. In severe, chronic cases an end-stage kidney develops. Infection is often ascending, originating in the lower urinary tract and is particularly likely when urinary stasis occurs, due either to obstruction of the urinary tract or paralysis of the bladder.

Cystitis: Inflammation of the bladder may be acute or chronic. In acute cystitis the mucosa is thickened and hyperaemic; the urine contains viscid exudate. In the cat there may be marked haemorrhage into the bladder. In chronic cystitis the bladder wall is thickened and the mucosal surface roughened, but hyperaemia is less marked. In follicular cystitis, nodules of chronic inflammatory cells are visible as small pale foci in the mucosa. Low grade cystitis may be present in the absence of clinical signs.

Neoplasia: Tumours of the bladder include tumours of the epithelium and of the muscle wall. Papillomas are not uncommon in dogs. Carcinomas are both locally invasive and frequently metastasize. Leiomyomas are ususally seen in dogs and, depending on their size and site, may cause urinary obstruction.

Male Genital System

Prostatic hyperplasia: This is a common change of old age in entire dogs. Enlargement may be considerable but is usually uniform. The structure is fairly normal but small cysts or foci of inflammation may occur.

Prostatitis: Areas of suppuration are obvious within an enlarged gland. Abscesses may cause irregular enlargement.

Neoplasia: The organ may be greatly enlarged and irregular. There is often invasion of local tissues. The tumour tissue is pale and solid and lacks normal structire.

Atrophy: In old dogs, senile atrophy occurs. The testes are small and composed of light brown, flabby tissue.

Orchitis: Small areas of congestion and necrosis may occur. Fibrosis may occur later.

Testicular neoplasia: Three types of tumour occur. They vary in appearance and significance. Tumours of more than one type may coexist. A small proportion of each type may be malignant and metastasize.

> **Seminoma:** These are composed of soft, cream-coloured tissue and may cause obvious enlargement of the affected testis which is the main clinical effect. Bilateral tumours are not uncommon.

> **Interstitial cell tumours:** They rarely cause enlargement of the affected testis and are usually of little significance. They are yellow/brown in colour and may contain areas of necrosis or cyst formation.

> **Sertoli cell tumours:** These are often not large and the affected testis is of normal size. The contralateral testis may be reduced in size due to hormone production by the tumour. The tumours are firm, white and often cystic and occur particularly in cryptorchid testes.

Female Genital Tract

Ovarian lesions: These include cysts of ovarian or paraovarian structures, and tumours. The latter may also be cystic, may be very large, and may be benign or malignant.

Uterine diseases: These include the cystic endometrial hyperplasia-pyometra complex and smooth muscle tumours. The endometrial lesions vary from cystic hyperplasia of the endometrium of enlarged uterine horns, to pyometra with an enlarged, thin walled uterus, containing mucopurulent fluid. Leiomyomas are common in the uterus and vagina, and may be large. Malignant tumours are rare.

ADDITIONAL INFORMATION

FURTHER READING

MOULTON, J.E. (1978). *Tumours in Domestic Animals.* 2nd Edition. University of California Press.

BOSTOCK, D.E. and OWEN, L.N. (1975). *A Colour Atlas of Neoplasia in the Cat, Dog and Horse.* Wolfe Medical Publications Ltd.

PETRAK, M.L. Editor (1969). *Diseases of Cage and Aviary Birds.* Lea Febiger, Philadelphia.

BENIRSCHKE, K., GARNER, F.M. and JONES, T.C. Volumes 1 & 2 (1978). *Pathology of Laboratory Animals.* Springer-Verlag, New York and Berlin.

JUBB, K.V.F., KENNEDY, P.C. and PALMER, N. Volumes 1 & 2, 3rd Edition (1985). *Pathology of Domestic Animals.* Academic Press, New York and London.

The following offer a diagnostic histopathology service for Veterinary Surgeons:
Abbey Veterinary Services, 7 Hopkins Lane, Newton Abbot, Devon, TQ12 2EL.
The Animal Health Trust, Balaton Lodge, Snailwell Road, Newmarket, Suffolk CB8 7DW.
Bloxham Laboratories, 5 George Street, Teignmouth, Devon TQ14 8AU.
Compton Paddock Laboratories, PO Box 91, Newbury, Berkshire RG16 0HB.
Diagnostic and Analytical Services, Chester Enterprise Centre, Hoole Bridge, Chester CH2 3NW.
J. Peter Finn, The Grange, Weybread, Diss, Norfolk IP21 5TU.
Grange Laboratories, PO Box 4, Wetherby, Leeds LS22 5JU.
Hoyward Ltd, 5 Hursley Road, Chandlers Ford, Eastleigh, Hants SO5 2FW.
Lab Pak Laboratories, 661 Foleshill Road, Coventry CV6 5JQ.
Leeds Veterinary Laboratories Ltd, Unit 3 Westfield Mills, Kirk Lane, Yeadon, Leeds LS19 7LX.
North Western Laboratories Ltd, Aldon Road, Poulton-le-Fylde, Blackpool, Lancashire FY6 8JL.
Vet Diagnostics, Victoria House, Small Dole, Henfield, Sussex BN5 9XE.
VetLab Services Ltd, Unit 11, Station Road, Southwater, West Sussex RH13 7HQ.
University Veterinary Schools.

INDEX OF LABORATORY EQUIPMENT SUPPLIERS

LABORATORY EQUIPMENT SUPPLIERS

The appended list of laboratory suppliers is not comprehensive and may not include all the products supplied by the firms listed. Telephone numbers are given so that when there is doubt, enquiries can be made.

The names of the various commercial laboratories supplying a service to veterinary practitioners are not included here but many can be found at the end of the section on post mortem examinations (page 143).

Product abbreviations

- A. General laboratory equipment suppliers.
- B. Specific haematological equipment.
- C. Specific clinical chemistry equipment.
- D. Blood collection/storage tubes and bottles.
- E. Stains, dyes and chemicals.
- F. Blood coagulation reagents.
- G. Urine analysis kits.
- H. Urine calculi kits.
- I. Serological/immunological reagents*.
- J. Clinical chemistry kits.
- K. Cytospin equipment.
- L. Swabs and transport media.
- M. Anaerobic jars or envelopes.
- N. Antibiotic sensitivity discs.
- O. Bacteriological culture media (various).
- P. Bacteriological containers and plates.
- Q. Disposable laboratory ware.

*Specialist laboratories often produce their own antisera for specific assays.

ADDRESSES

Products

Aldrich Chemical Co. Ltd.
The Old Brickyard, New Road, Gilingham, Dorset SP8 4JL
Telephone: 07476 2211 or 0800 717181 (orders)

A, E

Ames Division, Miles Laboratories Ltd.,
Stock Court, Stoke Poges, Slough SL2 4LY
Telephone: 02814 5151

G

API-bio Merieux (UK) Ltd.
Grafton Way, Basingstoke, Hampshire RG22 6HY
Telephone: 0256 461881

M

B.C.L. Ltd.
Boehringer Mannheim House, Bell Lane, Lewes, East Sussex BN7 1LG
Telephone: 0273 480444

B, C, D,
F. G, I, J

B.D.H. Chemicals Ltd.
Broom Road, Poole, Dorset BH12 4NN
Telephone: 0202 745520

E

Becton Dickinson UK Ltd.
York House, Empire Way, Wembley, Middlesex HA9 0PS
Telephone: 01-903 6544

B, D, M

Cambridge Research Biochemicals
Button End, Harston, Cambridge CB2 5NX
Telephone: 0223 871674

E, I

Camlab Ltd.
Nuffield Road, Cambridge CB4 1TH
Telephone: 0223 62222

D

Clandon Scientific Ltd.
Lysons Avenue, Ash Vale, Aldershot, Hants GU12 5QR
Telephone: 0252 514711

B

Coulter Electronics Ltd.
Northwell Drive, Luton, Beds. LU3 3RH
Telephone: 0582 491414

B

Diamond Diagnostics Ltd.
Mast House, Derby Road, Bootle, Merseyside L20 1EA
Telephone: 051 933 7277

N

Difco Laboratories
PO Box 149, Central Avenue, West Molesey, Surrey KT8 0SE
Telephone: 01 979 9951

I, O

Flow Laboratories
Woodcock Hill, Harefield Road, Rickmansworth, Herts WD3 1PQ
Telephone: 0923 774666

O

Gallenkamp
Belton Road West, Loughborough, Leics. LE11 0TR
Telephone: 0509 237371

A

General Diagnostics, Organon Teknika Ltd.
Science Park, Milton Road, Cambridge CB4 4BH
Telephone: 0223 313650

F

Gibco Ltd.
PO Box 35, 3 Washington Road, Paisley PA3 4EF
Telephone: 041 889 6100

I

ADDRESSES   Products

Gurr Stains, BDH Chemicals Ltd.
Broom Road, Poole BH12 4NN
Telephone: 0202 745520   E

Hawksley & Sons Ltd.
Malborough Road, Lancing, West Sussex BN15 8TN
Telephone: 0903 752815   B

Hughes & Hughes Ltd.
Elms Industrial Estate, Church Road, Harold Wood, Romford, Essex RM3 0HR
Telephone: 0402 349071   Q

ICN Biomedicals Ltd.
Lincoln Road, Cressex Industrial Estate, High Wycombe, Bucks HP12 3XJ
Telephone: 0494 443826   I

Kodak, Clinical Products Division Kodak Ltd.
PO Box 66, Station Road, Hemel Hempstead, Herts. HP1 1JU
Telephone: 0442 61122   C

Medical Wire and Equipment Co. Ltd.
Corsham, Wiltshire SN13 9RT
Telephone: 0225 810361   K, L

Merck Diagnostics UK agent, see BDH Chemicals Ltd. H

Oxoid Limited
Wade Road, Basingstoke, Hampshire RG24 0PW
Telephone: 0256 841144   N, O

Roche Products Ltd.
PO Box 8, Welwyn Garden City, Herts AL7 3AY
Telephone: 0707 328128   O

Sarstedt Ltd.
68 Bolton Road, Beaumont Leys, Leicester LE4 1AW
Telephone: 0533 359023   B, D

Shandon Instruments Ltd.
93—96 Chadwick Road, Astmoor, Runcorn, Cheshire WA7 1PR
Telephone: 0928 566611   K

Sigma Chemical Company Ltd.
Fancy Road, Poole, Dorset BH9 7NH
Telephone: 0202 733114 or 0800 373731 (orders)   E, J

Sterilin Limited
Lampton House, Lampton Road, Hounslow, Middlesex TW3 4EE
Telephone: 01 592 2468   D, P

Teklab (Medical Laboratories) Ltd.
9 Dorothy Terrace, Sacriston, Co. Durham DH7 6LG
Telephone: 091 371 0451   D

Trio Diagnostics
Thanet Industrial Studios, Albert Street, Ramsgate, Kent CT11 9HD
Telephone: 0843 583904   C

Vetlab Services Ltd.
Unit 10, Station Road, Southwater, Horsham, West Sussex RH13 7HQ   A. B. C.
Telephone: 0403 730176   D, L, M

Wellcome Diagnostics
Temple Hill, Dartford DA1 5AH
Telephone: 0322 77711   I

DESPATCH OF PATHOLOGICAL SPECIMENS BY POST

1. In general the despatch of deleterious substances by post is banned by the Post Office. There are, however, special exemptions for pathological material sent to and from laboratories by veterinary surgeons and some others. Very highly infected material, such as that containing foot and mouth disease virus or some especially dangerous human pathogens, are excluded from this exemption.

2. Members of the public may send specimens through the post only at the express request of a registered laboratory or veterinary surgeon.

3. Only **first-class letter post or data post** may be used. Parcel post must not be used.

4. The Post Office requires that all samples be packed in a particular way. These rules must be followed otherwise the Post Office may remove and destroy the specimen.

    (a) Every specimen must be enclosed in a primary container which is securely sealed. This container must not exceed 50 ml (although special multi-specimen packs may be approved).

    (b) The primary container must be wrapped in sufficient absorbent material to absorb all possible leakage in the event of damage.

    (c) The container and absorbent material must be sealed in a leakproof plastic bag.

    (d) This package must then be placed in either:
        (i)   A polypropylene clipdown container;
        (ii) A cylindrical light metal container;
        (iii) A strong cardboard box with full depth lid;
        (iv) A specially grooved two piece polystyrene box.

5. It is recommended that this completed package should then be placed in a padded bag.

6. Multi-specimen packs may be used provided that each primary container is separated from the next by absorbent packing.

7. Any other packaging systems must have prior approval of the Post Office.

8. (i) **Labelling:** The outer cover must be labelled 'Pathological Specimen — Fragile. With Care'. It must show the name and address of the sender to be contacted in case of leakage.
    (ii) It is important to record a unique identity on every sample (i.e. owner's name, animal identity) and the nature of the sample should also be noted (i.e. fixed tissue, heparin plasma, etc.)

9. Therapeutic and diagnostic substances, such as blood, serum, vaccines etc. are classified as pathological specimens.

Please be sure that anything you send by post complies with the regulations otherwise it may be removed from the mail and destroyed, and you will lose a valuable specimen. You may also be prosecuted by the Post Office. Even more importantly, you may cause injury or disease to someone handling the package either during its transit through the mails, or at the receiving laboratory.

LIST OF B.S.A.V.A. PUBLICATIONS

THE JOURNAL OF SMALL ANIMAL PRACTICE

An International Journal Published Monthly
Editor W. D. Tavernor, B.V.Sc., Ph.D., F.R.C.V.S.
Fifteen Year Cumulative Index published 1976

Available by post from
B.S.A.V.A. Registration Office
5 St. George's Terrace, Cheltenham, Gloucestershire, GL50 3PT

Manual of Exotic Pets
Revised Edition
Edited by
J. E. Cooper, BV,Sc., D.T.V.M., M.R.C.V.S., F.I. Biol.
and M. F. Hutchison, B.Sc., B.V.M.S., M.R.C.V.S.
assisted by
O. F. Jackson, Ph.D., F.R.C.V.S.
and R. J. Maurice, B.V.M.&S., M.R.C.V.S.
B.S.A.V.A Publications Committee 1985

Manual of Canine Behaviour
Valerie O'Farrell, Ph.D., A.B.P.S., (Clinical Psychologist)
B.S.A.V.A. Publications Committee 1986

Manual of Parrots, Budgerigars and other Psittacine Birds
Edited by C. J. Price, M.A., Vet.M.B., M.R.C.V.S.
B.S.A.V.A. Publications Committee 1988

Manual of Laboratory Techniques
New Edition
Edited by D. L. Doxey, B.V.M.&S., Ph.D.,M.R.C.V.S.,
and M. B. F. Nathan, M.A., B.V.Sc., M.R.C.V.S.
B.S.A.V.A. Publications Committee 1989

Manual of Anaesthesia for Small Animal Practice,
New Edition
Edited by A. D. R. Hilbery, B.Vet.Med., M.R.C.V.S.
B.S.A.V.A. Publications Committee 1989

Manual of Radiography and Radiology in Small Animal Practice.
Edited by R. Lee, B.V.Sc., D.V.R., Ph.D., M.R.C.V.S.
B.S.A.V.A. Publications Committee 1989

Manual of Small Animal Neurology
Edited by S. J. Wheeler, B.V.Sc., Cert.V.R., Ph.D., M.R.C.V.S.
B.S.A.V.A. Publications Committee 1989

B.S.A.V.A VIDEO 1 (VHS and BETA)
Radiography and Radiology of the Canine Chest
Presented by R. Lee, B.V.Sc., D.V.R., Ph.D., M.R.C.V.S.
Edited by M. McDonald, B.V.M.S., M.R.C.V.S.
B.S.A.V.A. Publications Committee 1983

Practical Veterinary Nursing
Second Edition
Edited by C. J. Price, M.A., Vet.M.B., M.R.C.V.S.
B.S.A.V.A. Publications Committee 1987

A Guide for Receptionists in Veterinary Practice,
Second Edition
Edited by N. R. Burton, B.V.Sc., Ph.D., M.R.C.V.S.
B.S.A.V.A. Publications Committee 1985

Aids to Nursing Small Animals and Birds,
Edited by J. S. Heath, M.R.C.V.S.
Ballière, Tindall & Cassell 1970

AVAILABLE FROM BOOKSELLERS

Canine Medicine and Therapeutics,
Second Edition
Edited by E. A. Chandler, B.Vet.Med., F.R.C.V.S.
Blackwell Scientific Publications 1984

An Atlas of Canine Surgical Techniques
Edited by
P. G. C. Bedford, Ph.D., B.Vet. Med., F.R.C.V.S., D.V.Ophthal
Blackwell Scientific Publications 1984

Jones Animal Nursing
Fourth Edition
Edited by D. R. Lane, B.Sc., F.R.C.V.S.
Pergamon Press 1985

Feline Medicine and Therapeutics
Edited by E. A. Chandler, B.Vet.Med., F.R.C.V.S.
C. J. Gaskell, B.V.Sc., Ph.D., D.V.R., M.R.C.V.S.
and A. D. R. Hilbery, B.Vet.Med., M.R.C.V.S.
Blackwell Scientific Publications 1985